Beyond a Glass of Milk and a Hot Bath

Advanced Sleep Solutions for People with Chronic Insomnia

By Connie Strasheim

About the Author

Connie Strasheim is a medical researcher and writer. She is the author, co-author or ghostwriter of 14 books on Lyme disease, cancer, nutrition, detoxification, sleep, mental health and spiritual healing. She collaborates with some of the world's finest integrative doctors in the writing of her books.

In addition, Connie is a prophetic healing prayer minister and passionate follower of Jesus Christ. She loves helping people with complex chronic illnesses to find freedom from disease and soul-spirit sickness using whole body medicine, miracles and prayer.

To learn more about Connie and her work, see: ConnieStrasheim.org

Contents

Chapter One

My Story and Why There Is Hope for You

If you have picked up this book, it's probably because you struggle to get enough quality shut-eye. It may feel like an agonizing battle, if the insomnia, or restless sleep, has lasted for months or years. If you're like me, you've probably tried many sleep medications, and gone to great lengths to try to get a good night's rest. Perhaps you have purchased sleep programs, enlisted the help of multiple health care practitioners, done sleep studies, and still—you seldom get a solid seven, eight or nine hours of sleep. Maybe you can't fall asleep, or you awaken frequently throughout the night. Or maybe you do sleep, but you awaken exhausted, because your sleep is light and unrefreshing. Whatever your sleep issues are, rarely do you feel rested when you awaken in the morning...or the afternoon, or whenever you do get up.

If this is you, I can relate! In fact, I'd like to share about my own battle with insomnia with you because I believe that it will give you hope. Once you read my story, and discover how I found my way out of the pit of sleeplessness, I believe you'll be inspired and encouraged to believe that there is a way out for you, too.

Insomnia was my wicked companion for years. It stole many years of my life, painted my world in shades of grey, and kept me from functioning and participating in society. It devastated my energy, filled my body with pain, distorted my thinking, and plummeted me into severe depression. At times, I wouldn't sleep for more than a few hours a night for weeks, especially during the two years when I was withdrawing from over a decade of benzodiazepine use.

During such times, I would sob and beg God for answers. When I wasn't doing that, I was either crying on the phone to a friend in the middle of the night because I couldn't sleep, or binging on oatmeal and carbohydrate-rich foods at 3 AM. Insomnia affected my relationships, severely disrupted my ability to function, and devastated my hope, my happiness and my livelihood.

It's not that I couldn't endure a night or two of sleeplessness here and there. Most of us can tolerate that. But insomnia relentlessly tortured me for years and turned me into an angry, whacked out, nearly non-functional human being. And at times when I was so sleep deprived that I thought that *surely* I would sleep the following night, I would not sleep at all. There were times when I actually wondered if I would die from sleep deprivation.

The reasons that I battled a severe sleep disorder were numerous. Foremost was the fact that I'd contracted a devastating neurological illness in my late 20's called Lyme disease. The infections involved in Lyme disease damaged my brain and nervous system and caused most every other part of my body to malfunction. This resulted in a multitude of symptoms, including insomnia.

Even worse, I became addicted to anti-depressants and benzodiazepines (sedative drugs) for over 10 years. The medications helped me to sleep at times while I recovered from Lyme disease and were very helpful in the short term.

However, over the long run, they caused imbalances in my body's chemistry and worsened the insomnia.

At the same time, for years I lived in an environment of high electromagnetic fields (one of the foremost causes of insomnia today), which kept me from getting enough shut-eye. Finally, I was tormented by past trauma and a fear of not sleeping, which added to the problem.

Because of all these factors, my battle to overcome insomnia was difficult and long. I had to remove the array of physical, emotional and spiritual stressors that were ruining my sleep, but the good news is...I did! And because of that, I am now able to share with you some solutions that may help you to overcome *your* battle with insomnia or restless sleep. Some of these solutions are not found in other books on sleep, so even if you have read every book out there, you are likely to find some new answers here.

I often used to sleep anywhere from 2-5 hours per night, and sometimes less than that—for years. And I am not one of those people who can get by on five hours of sleep, especially since I was battling a neurological disease. I really need eight hours of sleep to feel well rested. Now, I routinely sleep 7-9 hours per night. Occasionally, I still have trouble sleeping, especially when I travel or am under extreme stress, but I no longer take sleep medication except for in emergencies when I travel, and nights of total sleeplessness are rare.

The process of healing your brain, body and emotions, remediating your sleep environment, and revamping your sleep habits can take time, but I will attempt to help to shorten the treatment runway for you by sharing in this book everything that I did to recover my brain and body and remediate my environment.

What's more, I will help you to prioritize the solutions in a manageable order so that you can decide what to try first, and what to try last. I will also provide you with some insights that will help you to discover why you struggle to sleep in the first place, so that hopefully, you won't waste a lot of time, energy and money on tools that don't work for you. Chances are, you won't need to do everything that I did to recover my sleep, but I believe that you'll find at least a few tools here that will help you, as well!

Millions of people worldwide aren't getting enough quality sleep, for many reasons. For those of us who battle difficult health conditions, such as neurological and neurodegenerative illnesses like Lyme disease, chronic fatigue syndrome, fibromyalgia, Alzheimer's, Parkinson's, and multiple sclerosis—among others, the typical advice and solutions that are given to us by our doctors, books and other sources of information don't always work. A warm glass of milk, a hot bath, or a bit of valerian root or melatonin, while helpful, just doesn't cut it for many of us. So while this book is for anyone who isn't getting enough good quality sleep, its focus is primarily upon advanced solutions for those for whom the more conventional advice hasn't worked, such as people with neurological conditions.

Within the pages of this short book, I believe that you will find new answers that will not only help you to recover your sleep, but also your health, happiness and sanity.

As a final note, this book isn't meant to provide in-depth information on all of the solutions that are presented here, but rather, an overview, so that you can do further research on those solutions that appeal to you, on your own.

Be encouraged though, I believe that there is something for everyone in here! If you haven't found answers through the resources that have been made available to you, chances are, you will find some here. May you be blessed in your healing journey!

Chapter Two

Revitalize Your Sleep by Removing Electromagnetic Pollution from Your Home

Electromagnetic Pollution: The Invisible Neurotoxin that Keeps You Awake at Night

Manmade electromagnetic fields (EMFs) are a foremost cause of insomnia and restless sleep for many people today. We are all awash in a sea of EMFs, which come from things such as Wi-Fi routers, cell phones, power lines, household appliances, smart meters, wall wiring, cordless phones and computers. This might surprise you, but EMFs can profoundly disrupt your body's bioelectric energy, stimulate your nervous system, and make sleep challenging.

I've found that electromagnetic pollution is one of those toxins that most people don't take seriously though, and don't believe to be a cause of their symptoms, because the effects of EMFs upon the body aren't always apparent. But they are one of the most dangerous invisible toxins that we are all exposed to.

Thousands of studies have linked excessive exposure to EMFs to a multitude of chronic degenerative diseases and symptoms, including chronic fatigue, cancer, depression, headaches, brain fog and...you guessed it—insomnia! The Bio Initiative Working Group, which is a group of scientists, researchers and public health policy professionals dedicated to researching and reporting on the effects of EMFs, has a website with links to studies that demonstrate the dangerous effects of EMFs upon the body.

In the Working Group's 2012 Bio Initiative Report, researchers reported that "...The most serious health endpoints that have been reported to be associated with extremely low frequency (ELF) and/or radiofrequency radiation (RFR) include childhood and adult leukemia, childhood and adult brain tumors, and increased risk of the neurodegenerative diseases, Alzheimer's and amyotrophic lateral sclerosis (ALS). Recent studies largely reinforce the potential risks to health (rather than reducing our concerns, or providing actual indications of safety)."

"...In addition, there are reports of increased risk of breast cancer in both men and women, genotoxic effects (DNA damage, chromatin condensation, micronucleation, impaired repair of DNA damage in human stem cells), pathological leakage of the blood–brain barrier, altered immune function including increased allergic and inflammatory responses, miscarriage and some cardiovascular effects."

Finally, the researchers report, "Insomnia is reported in studies of people living in very low-intensity RFR environments with WI-FI and cell tower-level exposures."[i]

Despite the overwhelming evidence that EMFs damage DNA and cause or contribute to all kinds of illnesses, governments worldwide (especially the United States government) have failed to create stringent enough regulations to safeguard the population against their effects.

What's more, the amount of EMFs in the environment increases exponentially every year, as telecommunications companies construct new cell phone and Wi-Fi towers and our world becomes increasingly wireless. And unless you live in a tent out in the middle of the wilderness, chances are, your living environment has what most building biologists would deem to be harmful levels of EMFs.

If you haven't before, I want you to seriously consider EMFs as a potential cause of your insomnia. I used to think that EMFs weren't such a big deal until I moved out to the country, where the electromagnetic fields were much lower, and I began sleeping better than I had in years.

Prior to that, my sleep had been disrupted by EMFs in nearly every place that I had lived. EMFs weren't the *only* reason why I wasn't sleeping; Lyme disease pathogens had shipwrecked my brain, nervous system and hormones, and one side effect of that was chronic inflammation and insomnia. But EMFs may have been the straw that broke the camel's back, and I didn't realize how much until I left the mess of electromagnetic fields and moved to the country.

I mention electromagnetic pollution at the beginning of this book because it's not an incidental problem that occasionally contributes to people's health issues; rather, it is often one of the biggest factors in illness and sleep deprivation, and studies show that insomnia is one of the most common symptoms of electromagnetic pollution.

The good news is, there *are* things you can do to lower the EMFs in your environment. Some of you who are reading this may be thinking, "Well I did things to lower the EMFs at my home and it didn't help." It may be that EMFs are not an issue for you, but EMF remediation can be a bit complex, so before you conclude that your environment is safe, or that EMFs are not causing you to lose sleep at night, I'd like you to reconsider whether you've actually properly evaluated and remediated your environment.

Even if you know that EMFs aren't the cause of your insomnia or restless sleep, it's good to know about them because these fields harm your body by disrupting its bioelectric field. Many integrative doctors and holistic health care professionals now consider EMF remediation a necessary component of health maintenance. For this reason, I urge you—whether you have other health problems or not—to reduce the amount of electromagnetic pollution in your environment. This will help you to avoid getting cancer or another EMF-related malady such as a neurological illness ten years down the road. We are all susceptible to the damaging effects of EMFs, but some of us will be affected sooner or more than others.

Simple Tools for Reducing the Electromagnetic Pollution in Your Home

EMF remediation can be a bit complex, so I'm going to simplify it by sharing with you only those tools that I've personally found to be most effective and easy to use. However, to get the most out of your remediation efforts, I highly recommend learning a little about EMFs and how they can affect your body and environment. Camilla Rees' book: *Public Health SOS: The Shadow Side Of The Wireless Revolution,* although a bit older (published in 2009) is one great source of information on this topic, as is building biologist Oram Miller's outstanding website and business, which is called Create Healthy Homes: CreateHealthyHomes.com. The site contains a wealth of

downloadable information on how to make your home
EMF-safe.

Next, you'll want to purchase an electromagnetic field
meter to measure the EMFs in your home environment. In
general, the meters that are used to measure electrical and
radio frequencies are different than those used to measure
magnetic fields, but there is one relatively inexpensive
combination meter, by Cornet, called the ED78S EMF RF
Electrosmog meter.   This meter measures all types of
electromagnetic fields, including high and low magnetic
fields, and electrical and radio frequencies. It is also
relatively accurate and easy to use, and a great value for the
price.

The meter provides a numerical readout of the fields, in
addition to indicator lights. In general and simple terms, a
reading that falls within the "green" zone is generally good
and means that the fields are low in the area that you are
measuring. A reading in the low yellow range isn't terrible
(but may cause symptoms in sensitive people), and
anything above that indicates that you are living in an
environment of insomnia-inducing EMFs. For information
on specific acceptable frequency ranges, I recommend
reading Dr. Rees' book, *Public Health SOS: The Shadow
Side Of The Wireless Revolution.*

Electrical, radio frequency and magnetic fields all affect the
body in different ways and require separate remediation
solutions. The good news is, there are a few free, easy to
implement solutions for reducing both electrical and
magnetic fields in your environment, and you may find
that by doing these things alone, you can get more restful
sleep. They include:

- **Turning off the circuit breakers in your bedroom and other rooms at night.** Harmful electrical fields are transmitted through the wall wiring, electronic devices and appliances. When you turn off the circuit breakers, you stop those fields from entering your bedroom through the walls and devices.

- **Turning off your Wi-Fi router and cell phone**. Also, unplug any cordless phones in the house. Get off your phone and computer at least two hours before bedtime. The light from these devices and the EMFs that they generate stimulate your nervous system and pineal gland, the latter of which is responsible for your body's sleep/wake cycle.

- **Place your bed against the wall(s) and/or in the rooms where the EMFs are lowest.** You'll want to measure the magnetic, radio frequency (RF) and electrical fields in all of your rooms to discover which rooms and/or areas have the least amount of electromagnetic pollution. You can use the Cornet meter for this. Take multiple readings in all areas of the room, and at different times throughout the day.

You might be surprised at how the intensity and range of EMFs can vary from room to room within the same house, and even from one area in a room to another. For example, I once lived in a condominium that had a huge power line that ran through my bedroom attic and which connected to an outdoor lamp that was mounted on the outside of the building. Before I moved in, I had measured the fields in the bedroom during the day and found that they were low, and so I thought that I would have no trouble sleeping there.

Well, I was wrong! When the lamp was switched on at night, high voltage low-frequency electromagnetic fields radiated from the power line, and my Gauss meter (which is another device used to measure magnetic and low-frequency electrical fields) registered "in the red." My body literally vibrated while I slept!

Needless to say, the frequencies from the power line kept me from getting deep, restorative rest. Fortunately, the EMFs in my office were low, so I ended up sleeping in a mattress in that room for many months, until I could move to a less polluted environment.

I have moved three times over the past ten years due to EMF pollution. This is why I recommend that you take a bit of time to learn about EMFs so that you know how to identify whether your environment is safe, and what you can do about it if not, so that you don't have to move multiple times, as I did.

Electromagnetic pollution, in combination with the other factors that I mentioned earlier, made it difficult for me to sleep. Once I figured out what I needed to do, I no longer succumbed to their effects, but it was a bit of a learning process for me to find solutions that truly worked. I'm hoping to shorten the runway for you by sharing with you the tools that I have found to be most helpful. There are, after all, many EMF shielding products and other gadgets out on the market, and lots of conflicting advice about which ones work best.

But first, I recommend that you turn off your Wi-Fi router, cordless and cellular phones, electronic devices and circuit breakers at night. Doing these things may be sufficient to lower the EMFs in your environment. If not, and you still aren't sleeping and/or your EMF device(s) show high readings (in the yellow to red range), you'll want to purchase some EMF shielding tools to further clean up your environment. Following I share a few of my favorites which I have found to be effective and easy to use.

EMF Shielding Products that Work

Your body regenerates during sleep, so it is especially important to sleep in a low EMF environment. It isn't ideal to live in a sea of high EMFs during the day, either, but unless you live out in the country or in a remote location, it is nearly impossible to avoid being immersed in these fields during the day. But if you can create a low-EMF sleep sanctuary for yourself, this will go a long way toward helping your body to rejuvenate and recover from the damaging effects of EMFs.

There are many EMF shielding products on the market; not all work well, some are confusing or difficult to use and require the aid of a building biologist, while others are exorbitantly expensive, or harmful if used inappropriately. For this reason, I will try to make things a little easier for you by recommending only a few products that I have found to provide the greatest broad-spectrum benefit.

First, the shielding products that are used to block or absorb electrical and radio frequencies are different than those used to block magnetic fields. Magnetic shielding of large areas is, as a general rule, more expensive and complicated than shielding your bedroom from electrical and radio frequencies.

To shield yourself from radio frequencies (RF) from microwave towers, your cell phone, Wi-Fi, smart meters and other high-frequency sources of radiation, I recommend purchasing a shielding canopy to drape over your bed. These canopies are generally made of cotton or another fabric and have silver and/or copper woven into them, to protect you from the EMFs. They look a lot like a mosquito net and can be either hung from your ceiling or draped over a canopy frame.

Canopies can be purchased online from stores that sell EMF shielding products, such as EMFSafetyStore.com and LessEMF.com. Canopies vary in their effectiveness, and given that increasingly high levels of radio frequencies are being released into the environment, I recommend getting one with the highest level of frequency protection that you can afford.

One canopy that I recommend and really like is made from Swiss Shield Naturell fabric, and shields up to 99% of all frequencies up to 10 GHz. To my knowledge, it provides one of the highest levels of RF protection available. These canopies can be pricey, at $1,500-$1,600 for a queen-sized canopy, but a lifetime of insomnia (and other potential ailments) is far more expensive. In addition, they are a one-time investment that I have found to be well worth it. For more information on the Swiss Shield Naturell canopy, visit the EMF Safety Store and scroll down the page until you see: "Naturell Bed Canopy":
http://emfsafetystore.com/" \l "canopies".

Less expensive options using other RF shielding fabrics are also available. Most of these are still acceptable and will provide you with some protection against radio frequencies. They can be found on Amazon and other online stores for as little as $800.

If you can't afford a canopy, you may want to consider purchasing the shielding material that is used to create the canopy and then make one yourself. You can get shielding material online at Amazon, as well as at the EMF Safety Store: EMFsafetystore.com, The EMF Safety Shop: LessEMF.com and other retailers.

Magnetic Field Solutions

The Cornet meter that I described earlier, or any type of Gauss meter, can be used to measure magnetic fields in the home. Magnetic fields are harmful to the body—just as electrical and radio frequency fields—and they come from power lines, appliances, wall wiring and smart meters (all of which also emit electrical fields). It's important to shield yourself from both the electrical and magnetic fields that come from these sources of EMF pollution. While you will need a separate remediation solution for each type of field, finding a way to protect yourself from both electrical and magnetic fields doesn't necessarily have to be complicated or difficult.

First, measure the magnetic fields in your home using the Cornet meter, or you can purchase a separate Gauss meter to do this, as well (you can get cheap Gauss meters that will give you a general idea about the level of magnetic fields in the environment, for about $35 at LessEMF.com). If you find that the higher fields are confined to just a few small areas in your home, you may be able to get by with using some material made from high magnetic permeability metal alloys, to cover the walls or area where the fields are coming from. This material can be purchased at a variety of online retailers, and you'll want to ask the vendor about how to use it, because if you set it up wrong, it can make the fields worse. If the fields cover a large area though (as they often do), the process becomes more complex and expensive.

That said, whenever I have been exposed to high magnetic fields in my bedroom, such as when I lived in the condo with the high-voltage power line, I have found that it's much easier to first try to find an area in my home where the fields are relatively low, and put my bed there—rather than trying to remediate a large area. Unless you live near a power line, chances are, you'll be able to find a few spots in your home where you can do this.

However, you may need to purchase magnetic shielding material if your meter indicates that the fields are high everywhere in your home. Any reading above 1 mG (milligaus) is too high for most sensitive people and 1 mG is the level at which negative biological effects in the body are generally thought to occur. The average person may be able to tolerate fields that are a bit higher than that, but in the long run, regularly exposing yourself to fields above 1 mG may be harmful.

If you live less than 500 feet away from a large power line (which emits both electrical and magnetic fields), you may find that the magnetic fields in your home will be quite high (over 1 mG), everywhere in your home. If so, it may be important for you to either move or purchase magnetic shielding to cover all of the walls of your home—which is likely to be a complicated and pricey endeavor. So I recommend living away from large power lines, whenever possible. Studies have shown that people who live within 600 feet of a power line are more susceptible to certain types of cancer, such as leukemia.

The EMF Safety Store and other online stores that sell electromagnetic shielding can often provide advice about the type of shielding that you'll need for your bed and home. So if any of this seems confusing to you, don't worry! Stores and businesses that sell EMF shielding, as well as building biologists, can often help you to figure out what you need. The International Institute for Building Biology and Ecology contains a short list of building biologists in a few states. For more information, see: http://hbelc.org/find-an-expert/environmental-consultants.

Smart Meters – A Stealth Cause of Sleeplessness and How to Protect Yourself Against Their Effects

I have interviewed over 100 integrative and holistic doctors in my career as a medical writer, and a handful of the doctors that I have interviewed have mentioned that they have witnessed a surge in sleep disorders since smart meters have been installed onto most homes. Smart meters, which are used to measure energy usage, periodically generate electromagnetic pulses that jolt the nervous system and disrupt the body's bioelectric field.

Smart meters emit frequencies from two sources: first, from the meter itself, and secondly, from the wall wiring in your home. There are two ways that you can protect yourself from the effects of smart meters. First, you can purchase shielding material to cover the walls through which the smart meter may be radiating. Smart meter shielding is available online from retailers such as The EMF Safety Shop and The EMF Safety Store.

Secondly, you can purchase Graham-Stetzer filters, which plug into the wall outlets and neutralize what's called "dirty electricity" or the electrical fields that radiate from the wall wiring into the room. A set of 25 Graham Stetzer filters is generally enough to shield a 1,000-1,500 square foot home, costs about $500-800, and is well worth it.

I noticed a significant difference in my sleep when I added Graham-Stetzer filters to my repertoire of EMF shielding solutions. If you can't afford to shield your entire home, you can purchase the filters individually for $35. Even two or three filters, placed in your bedroom, will help to reduce the EMFs in your environment and may help you to sleep better. You can purchase Graham-Stetzer filters at Stetzer Electric: www.StetzerElectric.com or Stetzerizer-US.com.

You can also shield the smart meter itself or try to have it removed by the electric company; the latter can be difficult, but is well worth a try. A few states like California allow you to replace your smart meter with the old analog ones.

There are many other EMF-shielding products out there: devices that you can attach to your circuit breaker box, computer, cell phone and other appliances; EMF shielding paint, clothing, curtains and other items. For the purposes of getting better rest at night, I recommend first and foremost purchasing a shielding canopy and Graham-Stetzer filters. They are relatively straightforward and easy to use, have a great track record of success, and give you the most "bang for your buck." I personally witnessed the most significant and positive changes to my wellbeing by using just these two tools alone.

Finally, I recommend visiting building biologist Oram Miller's site: CreateHealthyHomes.com for periodic updates on how to protect yourself against the upcoming

5G, which is the fifth generation of the worldwide cellular mobile communications network that is being rolled out in 2019-2020. Current EMF remediation tools are likely to be effective for protecting your body against some of the frequencies that will be emitted by the 5G network—but not all of them. Many scientists are very concerned about the harmful effects of 5G upon the human body, and building biologists are currently developing products and other solutions to mitigate its effects.

Once 5G is deployed in your area, I encourage you to not utilize Wi-Fi or any "smart" devices in your home, including your smart phone, if possible. Keep your phone in airplane mode and turn it on only to check messages and make short calls. Use Skype, a landline and a hardwired Internet connection as the primary means to communicate with your loved ones. If this sounds extreme, consider this: the cell phone radiation from 5G is expected to be up to 100 times greater than what current cell phone devices emit, and scientists believe its effects to be far more harmful than the frequencies emitted by the 3 and 4G networks.

The good news is, experts believe that scalar wave pyramids made from materials such as shungite and ormusite may be very helpful for modulating any harmful frequencies in your home, including those that come from 5G. The company Fresh and Alive makes one such pyramid called the Rest Shield. However, you'll need to remove the "smart" technologies from your environment as much as possible, in order for these to be most effective. For more information, see: https://www.freshandalive.com/.

Chapter Three

Sleep Deeper by Lowering Histamine and Inflammation

Excessive levels of histamine and inflammation can be major causes of insomnia, especially in people with chronic health conditions. Histamine is a neurotransmitter that is involved in your body's immune response and is produced when you have an allergic response to something.

People with autoimmune-like chronic health conditions such as Lyme disease, mold illness, chronic fatigue syndrome, multiple chemical sensitivities, lupus and fibromyalgia, are often allergic to many things: foods, chemicals in the environment and so on. It follows that such people have high levels of histamine as their bodies get stuck in a perpetual inflammatory or allergic response to things in the environment. The diseases themselves can also cause histamine overload and immune system over-activation, which results in inflammation.

High histamine levels and inflammation in turn cause sleep disturbances. If you don't believe me, consider the medication Benadryl, which is often recommended by doctors as an over the counter sleep aid to block and/or shut down the effects of histamine and aid in sleep.

Histamine release is also implicated in mast cell activation disorder or disease (often abbreviated MCAD), a condition in which the body overproduces mast cells, and which is common in those with chronic health conditions of all kinds. Mast cells release histamine and cytokines, or chemicals that cause widespread inflammation throughout the body. Evidence for this is found in a study published in *Oxford Medicine Online* in April 2013, which reveals that substantial amounts of histamine are contained in, and can be released by, tissue mast cells.

Lawrence Afrin, MD, an expert in MCAD, cites many health conditions that are the cause or effect of MCAD in his book, *Never Bet Against Occam: Mast Cell Activation Disease and the Modern Epidemics of Chronic Illness and Medical Complexity*. The list is amazingly long and includes just about every chronic health condition that you can think of. Further, some integrative doctors of late have been finding that many conditions are caused in part or made worse by mast cell activation disorder, including chronic fatigue syndrome, fibromyalgia, mold illness and Lyme disease—among others.

If you haven't been tested for MCAD and have undiagnosed symptoms or a chronic condition that you haven't been able to successfully treat with the means that have been made available to you, I highly recommend talking to your doctor about MCAD. Proper treatment for MCAD can shut down many symptoms caused by inflammation, including, you guessed it—insomnia. Even if the only symptom that you have is insomnia, consider that excessive levels of histamine might be keeping you awake at night.

In early 2016, after having been substantially healed from insomnia and Lyme disease, I was exposed to several types of dangerous mold, including stachybotrys, one of the most damaging molds there is. Around the same time, I took some homeopathic remedies that, along with the mold, caused a massive, systemic, inflammatory response in my brain and spinal cord—worse than anything that I had ever experienced from Lyme disease. The result was a multitude of symptoms, including profound fatigue, depression, brain fog, chest pain, neuropathy, dizziness, gait problems and trouble walking, and tingling in my spine. I endured these horrific symptoms and was once again nearly bedridden for half a year.

Around the time that this happened, I had actually been sleeping relatively well, though—about 7 hours per night on average. Little did I know that mast cell activation was yet keeping me from sleeping as soundly as I could have been. I knew this because once one of my doctors prescribed me some remedies for MCAD I began to sleep deeper and longer than I ever had before—up to nine hours some nights, and my symptoms were reduced by over 50% literally overnight, after months of having tried many other treatments.

First, my doctor prescribed me ketotifen, a compounded antihistamine medication with a very low side effect profile. He then gave me quercetin and a supplement that contains diamine oxidase, an enzyme that's involved in the metabolism and inactivation of histamine. Within a few days, I was a new person.

It seemed that the mold toxins and the overreaction of my immune system to the injections had caused me to develop MCAD—or had at least exacerbated an underlying MCAD condition. When my doctor shut down the production of histamine in my body with these supplements and medication, I felt infinitely better and began to sleep more soundly.

Tools for Reducing the Symptoms of High Histamine,
Inflammation and Mast Cell Activation Disorder

If you have allergies or a serious chronic health condition of any kind, consider asking your doctor about giving you a trial treatment for mast cell activation disorder (MCAD). If you have this condition, it can affect your ability to sleep, and according to Dr. Afrin in his book, *Never Bet Against Occam,* it affects more people and plays a bigger role in many disorders than doctors and researchers once thought. I also recommend Dr. Afrin's book for more information about how to diagnose and treat MCAD. It is full of case studies and a bit challenging for the layperson to read, but is one of the best resources out there for learning about this condition.

While ketotifen, quercetin and diamine oxidase were helpful for treating the MCAD and enabling me to get deeper, more restorative sleep, you may find that other natural supplements or medications are more beneficial for lowering your histamine levels. Ketotifen was, at the time of the writing of this book, only available through a few compounding pharmacies in the United States (such as Key Pharmacy in Washington state) but it may be more widely available elsewhere. Diamine oxidase and quercetin are both available at online health food stores.

What I like about ketotifen is that it is profoundly effective and, unlike other commonly known antihistamines like Benadryl, it isn't anticholinergic; that is, it doesn't block the action of the neurotransmitter acetylcholine in the central and peripheral nervous system. Some antihistamines do this, and it is why drugs like Benadryl have been associated with Alzheimer's and memory loss, since acetylcholine plays a vital role in memory and cognition.

What's more, it's not just a Band-Aid for symptoms. In fact, it may even be healing to the body. A pharmacist that I spoke with at Key Pharmacy believes that it actually helps to re-set proper mast cell production in the immune system and especially, the gut. However, this process can take many months; even a year or longer. Ketotifen also has a relatively low side effect profile. The only side effect that I experienced from it was an increased appetite, which the pharmacist told me is actually a sign that my gut was being healed.

Ketotifen has so far been for me one of those little miracles of medicine that has made a huge difference in my wellbeing.

That said, there is no "one size fits all" approach for controlling histamine and MCAD, so it's best to work with a doctor who understands it. For instance, Neil Nathan, MD and Wayne Anderson, ND, are two expert integrative medical doctors in northern California who understand MCAD and histamine release. Both contributed a
chapter to my 2016 book, *New Paradigms in Lyme Disease Treatment: 10 Top Doctors Reveal Healing Strategies that Work.* For more information, see: www.NewLymeTreatments.com.

Fortunately, I believe that as MCAD becomes increasingly recognized within the medical community, more and more integrative doctors will be testing and treating their patients for it.

Quercetin, which may be one of the better-known natural remedies for treating MCAD, is described in Dr. Afrin's book *Never Bet Against Occam*. In it, Dr. Afrin says, "It (quercetin) seems to result in reduced production of inflammatory mediators (e.g., leukotrienes and histamine). It may also serve as an inhibitor of tyrosine kinases and other regulatory proteins of interest in activated mast cells."[ii]

Dr. Afrin notes that quercetin chalcone may be more easily absorbed than other forms of quercetin. By itself, quercetin wasn't sufficient to quell my symptoms, but it may be a good start for some of you who are reading this, if you know that MCAD and histamine are a problem for you.

Other nutrients that have anti-histaminic properties include: vitamin C, magnesium glycinate, curcumin and holy basil, all of which are believed to help the body to metabolize histamine.

Curcumin, a bright yellow chemical produced by the Indian spice turmeric, has been well studied for its anti-inflammatory effects. In fact, it may be one of the most powerful natural anti-inflammatory substances there is, and studies show that it decreases histamine, in addition to a variety of other inflammatory mediators such as cytokines.

For instance, Sunil Pai, MD who is an expert researcher on the benefits of curcumin, states in an interview with Ty Bollinger in *The Truth About Cancer* documentary that curcumin has been shown in studies to shut down over 97 mechanisms of inflammation, and there are over 5,000 studies demonstrating the incredibly powerful effects of curcuminoids.[iii]

If you try curcumin, it is important to use a product that your body can use, as not all sources of curcumin are very bioavailable. It's also important to use one that has a reputation for effectiveness. One product that I like is Dr. Pai's Bosmeric-SR, which contains a patented combination of curcumin, boswellia (boswellia serrata) and ginger extract (zingiber officinale) product. This product also apparently has substantial research to prove its effectiveness. For more information, see: http://www.bosmeric-sr.com//.

According to Dr. Afrin in his book, *Never Bet Against Occam,* other medications that can be used to treat MCAD include an anti-depressant called doxepin; tricyclic antidepressants, and benzodiazepines. I am not a fan of drugs that can cause other problems in the body such as these but some medications may be an acceptable short-term solution for cases of severe MCAD. In any case, I recommend asking your doctor about other treatment options, if you suspect MCAD is a problem for you.

The Benefits of an Anti-Histamine Diet

 Finally, some people have found that following an anti-histamine diet helps to reduce inflammation in the body and can therefore be beneficial for restoring sleep. Following an anti-histamine diet involves avoiding foods that have high levels of histamine or which release histamine in the body. These include, but aren't limited to:

- Alcohol
- Pickled and canned foods (e.g., sauerkrauts)
- Fermented food

- Processed foods with preservatives and artificial ingredients
- Chocolate and cocoa based products
- Vinegar
- Wheat
- Most citrus fruits
- Aged cheeses
- Shellfish
- Nuts (especially walnuts and cashews)
- Legumes (e.g., beans and chickpeas)
- Tomatoes

Of course, some people will be more affected by these foods than others, so you'll want to gauge your individual response to them, as well as to any other allergenic foods.

Leftover beef, chicken and other forms of animal protein can also accumulate histamine, so if you know that you are sensitive to it, avoiding leftovers may be a good idea.

Avoiding high histamine and histamine-releasing foods can be profoundly effective for some people. Judy Tsafrir, MD, a psychiatrist from New York, writes on her website: http://www.judytsafrirmd.com/ about how adopting a low-histamine diet helped to improve her own symptoms, including insomnia.

Says Dr. Tsafrir, "I stopped eating left overs. I cooked smaller pots of food and froze the left overs in individual containers. I stopped eating cheeses, bacon and avocado. I began eating more salads. Most foods contain histamine, so you cannot have a histamine free diet like you can have a gluten free diet. But it is the relative quantity of histamine in relationship with your own capacity to handle it that translates into symptoms. I clearly was overwhelming my capacity to metabolize the histamine quantity that I was ingesting."

She then says, "Within days of instituting the dietary changes, I slept better than I have in years; very deeply and I dreamt. This is unusual for me. I have had insomnia since I was a child, probably due to life-long undiagnosed histamine intolerance. A sense of calm and peace replaced the chronic anxiety I was experiencing, my spirits lifted and I felt much less tired and more alert. Given the strength and immediacy of my response to lowering the histamine content of my diet, I believe that histamine intolerance should be considered in every case of anxiety disorder, depression, sleep and attention disorders, especially if a person is aware of food sensitivity issues."[iv]

To summarize, shutting down histamine and/or mast cell production can have profound positive and far-reaching benefits upon the body, and result in improved sleep. I never knew how much of a role histamine and MCAD was playing in my symptoms and sleep patterns until I began treating the issue. And I was amazed at how much deeper my sleep was when I did. If you suffer from any kind of chronic inflammatory condition that includes insomnia, I encourage you to consider histamine and MCAD as a possible cause.

Chapter Four

Replenish Your Neurotransmitters Naturally

Neurotransmitters are chemical messengers that coordinate the transmission of signals between nerve cells in your brain and throughout your body. They regulate a multitude of processes including emotions, memory, cognition, concentration, alertness, energy, appetite, pain, and of course—sleep.

Neurotransmitters affect every cell, organ and system in your body, and are linked to your immune and endocrine (hormonal) systems. This means that any imbalances and/or abnormalities can cause a variety of health problems, including insomnia.

Neurotransmitters can become imbalanced in the body due to stress, nutritional deficiencies, environmental toxicity and illness. Unfortunately, it's not uncommon for people nowadays to have deficiencies of the calming neurotransmitters that aid in sleep, and an excess of the excitatory ones that keep them awake.

I already shared about how histamine disrupts sleep, but another neurotransmitter that causes insomnia when found in excess in the brain and body is glutamate.

Reduce Glutamate, the Neurotransmitter that Disrupts Sleep

Glutamate is your brain's main excitatory neurotransmitter that plays a role in learning, cognition and memory. It is also the precursor for GABA, which is your brain's primary inhibitory, or relaxing, neurotransmitter.

Unfortunately, stress, a poor diet, illness and other factors can disrupt the glutamate-GABA conversion, and this, among other factors, can result in elevated levels of glutamate in the body. This translates into poor sleep, since glutamate is an excitatory, or stimulatory neurotransmitter that awakens the nervous system.

Over the long haul, excessive levels of glutamate lead to brain inflammation, neuronal destruction and ultimately, neurodegeneration. So while glutamate is essential for the brain, in excess it harms it. In fact, studies suggest that many neurodegenerative disorders such as autism, ALS and Parkinson's, are caused at least in part by glutamate excess.

Many people who battle neurodegenerative diseases have excessive levels of glutamate in their brain. Throughout my recovery from Lyme disease, my neurotransmitter test results consistently revealed that my glutamate levels were high, and my pharmacist believed that this was playing a role in my inability to sleep. At the time that I discovered this, I had already been using a couple of remedies to help me sleep, and while I had had some measure of success with these, I still wasn't getting a solid seven or eight hours every night, which is what I needed.

I told my pharmacist and he recommended that I take oxaloacetate, a compound that has been found to help decrease glutamate levels in the brain by activating an enzyme responsible for scavenging glutamate. One study, the results of which were published in *The Journal of Neurological Anesthesiology* in July 2009, showed treatment with oxaloacetate after traumatic brain injury to decrease blood glutamate levels and protect against the neurotoxic effects of glutamate on the brain.[v]

You can find oxaloacetate in a few online stores, in products such as Sabre Science's Cereze: http://www.sabresciences.com/store/ and benaGene http://benagene.com.

If neurotransmitter testing reveals that your glutamate is outside of the normal range, you may find that supplementing with oxaloacetate will help you to sleep. As a side note, it must be taken on an empty stomach, away from other supplements. One study published in *The Journal of Neurochemistry* in 2003 showed that large doses of oxaloacetate could reduce levels of glutamate by 30-40% in lab animals, which indicates that it is a potentially potent neuroprotectant and sleep aid.[vi]

While the results that I experienced from oxaloacetate weren't dramatic, I believe that it moved my sleep patterns another notch in the right direction. In any case, it is a useful supplement for helping to lower levels of this excitatory neurotransmitter and for protecting the brain against its toxic effects.

*Amino Acids That Support Sleep and Healthy
Neurotransmitter Production*

GABA

Perhaps the most important calming neurotransmitter
involved in sleep is GABA, or gamma-amino butyric acid.
GABA promotes restful sleep by decreasing neuron firing
in the brain. Its calming properties can also reduce anxiety
and balance blood pressure.

GABA is an amino acid in addition to a neurotransmitter,
and I have found GABA supplements to be one of the most
powerful tools for helping me and many other people to
overcome insomnia. By itself, GABA wasn't enough for me
but it has been one of the most important components of
my sleep protocol, and I continue to use it to this day.

Not just any regular ol' form of GABA worked for me,
though. I tried some GABA straight off of the supermarket
shelf and felt horrible the first morning after I took it. Little
did I know my body couldn't metabolize it well and I
needed to use a more bioavailable form. So for a long time,
I concluded that I didn't need GABA, until one day, I came
across a great product that a friend had urged me to try,
and which worked for me.

That product was Kavinace, made by NeuroScience. It
contains bioavailable GABA, in addition to taurine, which
is an amino acid that can also help to block the negative
effects of glutamate upon the brain. You may find that
Kavinace will work better for you than other GABA
products as well, especially if you have methylation issues
and genetic defects (more on this later) that prevent your
body from effectively utilizing amino acids. Kavinace costs

more than just plain ol' GABA, but it has made a world of difference in my wellbeing. If you haven't tried Kavinace, I encourage you to do so, especially if neurotransmitter testing indicates that you need GABA. It is one of the most powerful natural sleep aids there is.

You can purchase Kavinace at many online retailers such as: PureFormulas.com.

Taurine

Taurine is an amino acid that is found in high levels in the central nervous system. One of its roles is to help modulate and promote healthy levels of GABA. While taurine was not a core element of my sleep protocol, I found that by combining it with GABA, it improved my sleep at times when I needed just a little extra something to get by.

Another benefit of taurine is that it helps to prevent neuron damage caused by excessive levels of glutamate. Experimental studies on rats have shown that taurine inhibits glutamate toxicity through a number of different mechanisms.[vii] This is good news for those of us who suffer from cognitive and other brain symptoms caused by neurodegenerative diseases like Lyme. Taurine can be purchased at many online retailers and health food stores.

Theanine

Theanine, which is another calming amino acid, is also believed to play an important role in modulating several neurotransmitters, especially GABA. I personally found theanine to be less powerful and sedating than GABA, but some people prefer it to GABA.

You will most likely find that you will need to experiment to determine what types of products and amino acids that your body needs. Doing amino acid and neurotransmitter urine testing through a reputable lab (more on lab testing later) can be helpful, but even tests are imperfect and you and your doctor may need to experiment a little to discover what you will need.

Tryptophan and 5-HTP

While GABA, taurine and theanine are all fantastic calming amino acids that aid in sleep two others that you may benefit from in addition to, or instead of these, are 5-HTP and/or tryptophan. Me, I needed the whole kit n' caboodle. As crazy as that may sound, I had to do multiple things to restore my sleep, and while I have now narrowed my sleep supplements down to just two: cannabis (more on this later) and one combination product called Kavinace Ultra PM, which contains GABA, 5-HTP and melatonin— for awhile, I needed to use a variety of tools to "reboot" and restore my body.

Tryptophan and 5-HTP are amino acids that are both precursors to serotonin, which is another calming neurotransmitter that helps the body and mind to relax, and is a powerful mood promoter. Most of you have probably heard about 5-HTP and tryptophan, but what you may not know is that these amino acids don't always work that well in the body unless you have all of the proper co-factors and/or methylation support that your body needs to synthesize serotonin from them.

For instance, you may find that if you have any methylation issues or genetic defects (which are relatively common in today's toxic world) you may not benefit from taking these amino acids unless you have the proper methylators, and/or nutrients to make them work in your body. Methylation is a process that occurs in all of our cells and is a key biochemical process that is essential for the proper function of nearly all of our body's systems. One of its roles is to help us make neurotransmitters, but some of us have methylation problems that keep us from being able to do that.

Later in this section I describe some methylators/nutrients that you may find useful for helping your body to synthesize neurotransmitters from amino acids. You'll want to discuss these with your doctor and ideally, get tested to discover which ones you may benefit from. A few companies offer genetic testing that can provide insights into your body's ability to synthesize and break down neurotransmitters.

If you can't afford genetic or other types of testing, you can ask your doctor to give you a trial treatment of amino acid therapy, to see how you respond. This is less ideal, but can sometimes provide enough insight into what supplements you may need.

Some people have commented to me that they feel worse when they take amino acids. I have at times, too. This can be due to several factors. First, and as I just mentioned, your body may not be able to synthesize neurotransmitters from amino acids due to a methylation or other genetic problem. This means that your body won't use the amino acids properly and you will either experience no discernible benefit after taking them, or you will end up feeling worse.

Secondly, if you are highly deficient in certain amino acids and/or neurotransmitters, you can also feel worse when you first start amino acid therapy. If neurotransmitter testing reveals that you are deficient in certain neurotransmitters, you may want to ask your doctor to prescribe you low doses of the appropriate amino acid precursors, and then you can slowly work your way up on the dosing. Taking a dose that is too high, too soon, can make you feel worse.

The first time that I took a 5-HTP product I became more brain fogged, depressed and fatigued. I mistakenly concluded that amino acids were not helpful for me. Unfortunately, I continued to sleep poorly for several years after that, until I realized that the problem wasn't that my body didn't need 5-HTP, but rather, that it couldn't make serotonin from the 5-HTP without a little help. Once I discovered the nutrients and methylating substances that my body needed to synthesize serotonin from 5-HTP, I actually became more energetic, clear-headed, and happy— and my sleep improved.

You can purchase 5-HTP, tryptophan, theanine and all of the other amino acids described in this section at many health food stores and online retailers. Quality is likely to vary among the products, so it's a good idea to get one that has been recommended by a reputable health care practitioner. Personally, I have found the NeuroScience products to be most effective, but they are more expensive than some other amino acid products so they may or may not be the best option for you. To learn more about NeuroScience's products, see: NeuroScienceInc.com.

Methylators and Co-Factors Help the Body to Make
Neurotransmitters

As I mentioned, amino acids may not work properly in your body if you take the wrong product, dosage or combination of nutrients, or if you need methylators and/or nutritional co-factors, which assist in neurotransmitter synthesis. This is important to understand if you have tried amino acids before but not had good results from them.

I have found that many people, especially those who battle chronic neurological diseases may need methylation support, along with amino acids. Some common methylators that help the body to synthesize neurotransmitters from amino acids include:

- SAM-e
- Methyl-folate (a bioavailable form of folate)
- P5P (pyridoxyl phosphate, which is a bioavailable form of Vitamin B-6)
- Vitamin B-12

In addition, your body needs an adequate supply of zinc, magnesium, vitamin C and vitamin B-6 to make serotonin from 5-HTP, so if you are deficient in these nutrients, taking one or more of them may be helpful.

Ideally, to find out which methylators you may need, it's best to have your doctor do a complete amino acid and neurotransmitter profile, which are available through many labs and compounding pharmacies such as:

- Sabre Sciences (SabreSciences.com)
- NeuroScience (WhyNeuroScience.com)

- Pharmasan (Pharmasan.com)
- BioHealth Diagnostics (BioHealthLab.com)

In addition, you'll want to do a gene test, the results of which your doctor can use to determine whether you have genetic defects that hamper your body's ability to properly synthesize and metabolize neurotransmitters and other chemicals.

Again, if you can't afford lab testing, which can be expensive, and if your doctor approves, you might try a low trial dose of 5-HTP and/or GABA. If you don't notice that either amino acid improves your sleep or you feel worse after taking them, consider adding a small dose of SAM-e, P5P and/or methyl-folate, according to your lab results and/or doctor's recommendations. A small dose of SAM-e would be about 50 mg, taken in the morning (as it can disrupt sleep when taken at night). Again, even if you do lab testing, you may find that you need to experiment with the methylators and dosages to find the one(s) that will work best for you.

When I first started using methylators, I found that I could not tolerate more than half a capsule of SAMe. If I took more, it actually kept me up at night and worsened the insomnia. But a small amount helped my body to utilize the amino acids that I needed to get proper rest. I then introduced a small amount of P5P into my regimen, and finally, methyl-folate. I added them one at a time to gauge my response to each.

I highly recommend supplementing in this way and doing lab tests to determine what your body needs, as taking too much of any one methylator can actually cause your body to over-methylate, which can have an opposite effect and keep you up at night. In any case, it is always best to consult with a knowledgeable integrative doctor and/or compounding pharmacist for help in balancing your chemistry.

You may want to dose your amino acids in a similar fashion. Ask your doctor about starting with one, say, 50 mg 5-HTP capsule or tablet (maybe even half a 50 mg capsule) and then increasing the dose over time until you notice that you are sleeping better. Typical doses can range from 50 mg up to 300 mg, per your doctor's recommendations. You can also try L-tryptophan, which is the amino acid precursor to 5-HTP and also works well for some people.

Personally, I prefer 5-HTP because it is one step closer to serotonin on the neurotransmitter synthesis chain, which means that my body doesn't have to go through as many steps to create serotonin from 5-HTP as it does from tryptophan, and I tend to respond better to 5-HTP. However, some people find it more beneficial to take a combination of both 5-HTP and tryptophan.

One doctor who helped to treat my neurotransmitter dysfunction, Jeremy Kaslow, MD, who is an expert in neurotransmitter balancing, once told me that some of his patients fared best by taking both 5-HTP and tryptophan at bedtime. Dr. Kaslow has some great articles on neurotransmitter support. You can read about these at: http://drkaslow.com/html/neurotransmitter_repletion.html.

How to Determine Whether Amino Acid Therapy Is Right for You

First, if you take antidepressants, you'll want to consult with your doctor before taking 5-HTP or L-tryptophan, as these amino acids are sometimes contraindicated in those who use anti-depressants and the two remedies together can occasionally cause a condition known as serotonin syndrome. I have personally never met anyone who has had this problem, but it does exist, so if you are on an antidepressant, use amino acids with caution and only under the guidance of a qualified health care practitioner.

Also, serotonin and dopamine must both be balanced in the body in order for each to work optimally. Both neurotransmitters regulate mood and cognition, but dopamine is an excitatory neurotransmitter that also gives you energy.

The amino acid precursors to dopamine are L-phenylalanine and L-tyrosine. Both can increase energy, and in excess, cause anxiety and/or heart palpitations, and are best taken in the morning. Again, I recommend doing a complete amino acid and neurotransmitter profile to determine whether you might also benefit from L-tyrosine or L-phenylalanine. Neither of these plays a direct role in sleep but when all of your neurotransmitters are balanced in relationship to one another, everything functions better, including your sleep-wake cycle.

Finally, you may be asking how you can know whether neurotransmitter imbalances are causing your insomnia. That's a good question! I think the easiest way to find out, without doing extensive testing, is to do a trial treatment of amino acid therapy, and/or take an inventory of your mood, energy, pain levels, and sleep patterns and see how these change when you supplement with amino acids. If they are beneficial for you, you should notice positive changes in your mood, cognition, pain, energy, and of course—sleep.

I have found neurotransmitter imbalances to be a major cause of insomnia in many people, especially those with neurodegenerative diseases. For instance, chronic Lyme disease depletes neurotransmitters or leads to neurotransmitter imbalances, as do many other chronic health conditions. Also, if you have a history of childhood abuse or trauma, chances are, you have neurotransmitter imbalances, since trauma depletes the body of many chemicals, including amino acids and neurotransmitters.

In the end, the steps that you'll want to take to determine whether amino acid therapy is right for you, include:

1) Doing a complete amino acid and neurotransmitter profile through a reputable lab such as Sabre Sciences, NeuroScience, Pharmasan and/or BioHealth Diagnostics.

2) Doing a trial treatment of amino acid therapy to see if it is right for you. I always recommend doing this under a doctor's care, so that he/she can gauge your reactions to determine what you might need and how your regimen needs to be adjusted.

3) Supplementing with the appropriate co-factors that aid in neurotransmitter synthesis, such as zinc, magnesium and vitamin C (which are often depleted in people with chronic illness).

4) Supplementing with methylators that will help your body to make neurotransmitters from amino acids. (Take these only if your test results indicate that you need methylation support, you respond poorly to amino acids, and your doctor tells you that you need them).

Clues that you may have a methylation problem include: 1) Having a negative reaction or feeling worse when you take amino acids 2) Genetic testing indicates that you need methylation support or 3) Test results indicate that you have amino acid deficiencies but taking the appropriate amino acids seems to produce no change in your symptoms or ability to sleep.

5) The most commonly used methylators that aid in neurotransmitter synthesis include:

- SAM-e
- Vitamins B-6 (or pyridoxyl phosphate, P5P)
- Vitamin B-12 (methyl and/or adenosyl B-12 tend to be the most effective forms of these B vitamins). You may need one or more of these
- Methyl-folate

In addition, if your test results show that you have high levels of histamine and/or glutamate, consider:

6) Lowering your histamine levels with quercetin, a diamine oxidase product, and/or anti-histaminic medications

7) Lowering your glutamate levels by maintaining a gluten and casein-free diet, and supplementing with theanine and/or oxaloacetate.

Chapter Five

Modulate Your Brain Waves with Entrainment Therapy

Brain wave entrainment therapy is another neat tool that played a crucial role in my recovery from insomnia. It was especially useful for helping me to wean off of benzodiazepine and anti-depressant drugs. You may find it to be useful for restoring your sleep patterns, as well, and/or for helping you to get off of sleep medication.

One type of brain entrainment device that I found to be particularly helpful, called a neurofeedback device, uses feedback from your brain to modulate your brain waves, and in so doing, helps you to fall asleep at night. The neurofeedback device was especially useful for helping me to sleep when the drug withdrawal process made my insomnia even worse, and for helping me to stay the course when I was tempted to relapse and get hooked on the sleep meds again. It was one of the first, and most powerful tools that I used to recover my sleep.

I describe brain entrainment in my 2014 book, *BioEnergetic Tools for Wellness*, which I co-authored with integrative doctor Lee Cowden, MD, who is an expert in energy medicine. The therapy is described in the sections entitled *Neurofeedback* and *Light and Sound Machines*. Following are those excerpts for your convenience (*Taken*

*by permission from BioEnergetic Tools for Wellness ©
William Lee Cowden, MD and Connie Strasheim, 2014.)*

Neurofeedback

The neurofeedback device is a type of biofeedback device that measures your brain waves. It then uses that information to produce a signal that can be used as feedback to regulate your brain activity. Neurofeedback is an extraordinarily useful tool that can fully resolve or at least improve symptoms of insomnia in most people.

Unlike dangerous chemical sleep medications, such as benzodiazepines (sedatives), antidepressants and other drugs, which are often given in conventional medicine to treat insomnia, neurofeedback doesn't cause addictions or toxicity in the liver, or create long-term neurotransmitter imbalances or other undesirable side effects. Instead, it entrains your brain, or essentially teaches it, how to behave like it's supposed to at night. Over time, it can permanently alter your brain wave patterns and positively affect your brain chemistry.

Many studies have proven that neurofeedback has a strong track record of success at treating a variety of neurological conditions, not just insomnia. For instance, it has proven to be useful for reducing symptoms of autism, epilepsy, headaches, depression, anxiety and brain damage from strokes.

Many of us have had a head and/or brain injury sometime during our lifetime, but we may or may not have been aware of it. For instance, we may have had a prolonged or difficult birth, which damaged our brain in some way, unbeknownst to us. Quantitative EEG mapping tests have also proven that some viruses, microbes and toxins can cause brain damage patterns similar to those of physical traumas, such as when a person is dealt a blunt blow to the head.

Brain injuries can contribute to insomnia, anxiety, depression, impaired concentration and/or memory, difficulty with problem solving, and other neurological issues. Neurofeedback is excellent for repairing such damage, and thereby mitigating symptoms.

Neurofeedback can be done in a clinic, but some companies also sell neurofeedback devices that you can use at home. The one that I used had sensors that were attached to leads, which I placed on strategic locations on my head. The leads provided feedback to the device about my brain wave patterns. The device then used this feedback as input to normalize those patterns, and subsequently, my brain function, so that I could sleep when I was supposed to sleep, and remain awake when I was supposed to be awake.

The type of neurofeedback system that I used, and which has a strong track record of success is called the Neurointegrator, which is made by Clear Mind. To use the Neurointegrator, I simply put on a pair of glasses with blinking lights at bedtime, along with the sensors and leads, while I closed my eyes and listened to music. I usually fell asleep sometime during the 45-minute treatment.

The Clear Mind website has a link to studies which show that the Clear Mind neurofeedback programs have an 80 percent success rate at reducing or eliminating symptoms of insomnia (as well as some other neurological conditions such as anxiety and depression).

Clear Mind treatments can also be done at a clinic. These are more powerful and might cost an average of $100 to $150 per session. At the time of the writing of this book, the personal device that I used at home (the Neurointegrator) was available for approximately $3,500. The Clear Mind company also now makes a device called the Focus Unit, which uses a somewhat different brain wave technology to restore sleep. It is described later in this section.

Severe cases of insomnia may require 50 or more nightly neurofeedback treatments (especially if you have been addicted to benzodiazepines), so it's worthwhile to invest in a home unit if you can afford it, rather than go to a clinic that offers treatments.

Alternatively, and if your funds are tight, you may want to try a light-sound device, which is another type of brain wave entrainment therapy that can be just as effective as neurofeedback, but which costs much less. It is described in the following section.

I was drawn to Clear Mind after one of the Clear Mind Center's company representatives shared with me that his wife had been taking the sleep medication Ambien for 15 years, but found that she was able to completely wean off of it once she started using the brain entrainment device. That inspired me to purchase a sleep device for myself, as, at that time, I had been weaning off of benzodiazepines and was sleeping as little as 2-3 hours some nights. The device was a financial sacrifice for me, but one that I found to be well worth it to get my sleep and sanity back. As I mentioned, I needed other tools to fully restore my sleep patterns, but the Neurointegrator device gave me a huge push in the right direction.

As I mentioned earlier, you may or may not need as many tools as I did to recover your sleep. I had a lot working against me, including Lyme disease, many years of sleep medication use, and a history of trauma—among other issues, so my recovery required that I use more than just a couple of tools to get well. But by "stacking" those tools, I eventually healed my neurological system to a significant degree. However, you may find just one tool, such as a brain entrainment device, or amino acid therapy, to be enough for you.

For more information on Clear Mind brain entrainment devices, or to find a practitioner in your area that does Clear Mind treatments, see the Clear Mind website: ClearMindCenter.com.

Light and Sound Machines

Light and sound machines are another type of brain entrainment device that modulates your brain wave patterns to help you sleep at night. Light and sound machines feed-in fixed energetic frequencies to your brain, rather than utilizing feedback from your brain to adjust your brain wave frequencies, as neurofeedback devices do.

Basically, light and sound machines utilize pre-programmed brain wave pattern protocols to deliver energetic frequencies to your brain. They do this with the aid of blinking-light glasses, and/or audio sounds which are delivered to your eyes and ears through a set of headphones. Using these frequencies, the light and sound machine gradually entrains your brain into a slow delta-wave pattern, which is what your body needs for deep sleep.

Of the many therapies that Dr. Cowden has used on his patients over the years, he has found the light and sound machine to be one of the best for resolving insomnia. Some people prefer to use only the sound component of the device for sleep, while others prefer to use only the light component. Fortunately, both of these can be effective by themselves, although it's preferable to use both the sound and light components together for best results.

Most of these types of devices start by entraining your brain at a higher frequency, and then slowly ramp down on the frequencies until your brain effectively reaches a delta wave frequency. So, for instance, the device might start by entraining your brain at a beta frequency of around 30 Hz. (Your brain is in a beta state when you are fully awake and alert).   Over a few minutes, the device will then slowly ramp down your brainwave frequencies into the alpha range; say, 8 to 13 Hz. The alpha waves put your brain into a more relaxed state. Then, the device will ramp down your brainwave frequencies even further, into the theta range; say, 5 to 7 Hz, and finish the program in the delta frequency range, which is about 1 to 4 Hz.

By the time you get down into the 1 to 4 Hz range, you should be asleep. Both the flashing lights on the glasses and the audio sounds function to slowly bring your brain into this delta wave pattern.

One advantage of light and sound machines is that they are relatively affordable, compared to some other types of brain entrainment therapies, such as the Clear Mind neurofeedback device. You can purchase a good light and sound machine for anywhere from $159 to $600 on websites such as: ToolsForWellness.com.

Chapter Six

Balance Your Hormones with Supplements and Bio-Identical Hormone Replacement Therapy (BHRT)

Few things disrupt sleep as much as hormonal imbalances, which are caused by many things, including environmental toxins, illness, stress, a poor diet and simply aging.

Hormonal imbalances are very common in our toxic world, and if you are battling a chronic illness, chances are, your hormones are even more out of whack. Many people today have adrenal dysfunction, which results in an underproduction or overproduction of adrenal hormones. This condition occurs when there is a constant drain on the body from stress, inflammation, sickness, environmental toxicity and other factors. And one major symptom of adrenal dysfunction is insomnia.

Similarly, many of us are suffering from suboptimal thyroid function, which is caused by many of the same factors as adrenal fatigue. For instance, environmental contaminants such as fluoride are widely known to damage the thyroid. And in fact, adrenal fatigue often leads to thyroid hormone imbalances and vice versa.

I had a stressful upbringing and spent most of my life living in fear, or "fight-or-flight" mode. This, along with battling chronic Lyme disease and being exposed to all kinds of environmental contaminants burned out my adrenal glands and caused my thyroid to malfunction. Because both the thyroid and adrenals affect sleep, another step in my healing process involved restoring hormonal balance to my body.

It wasn't easy, and to this day, my adrenal and thyroid function are not perfect, because I've had a lot of major stressors to overcome since I first became sick in 2004. The good news is, my health has improved enough to where I am able to function and sleep well most nights, even though my adrenal and thyroid function remain less than optimal. But I had to address the health of my adrenal glands and thyroid to some degree in order to recover my sleep. You may find that you need to do the same, especially if you have a chronic health condition or are a woman over the age of 35.

You may know that balancing the hormones can be challenging, and I have found that few health care practitioners really know how to do it well, especially in those of us who have battled serious chronic neurological or autoimmune-like illnesses like Lyme disease, fibromyalgia, Parkinson's, Multiple Sclerosis or chronic fatigue syndrome. The good news is that if you are addressing all of the other factors that are contributing to your lack of sleep, you don't necessarily have to have perfect hormonal balance.

It is beyond the scope of this book to describe in detail every strategy for balancing the hormones, or endocrine system, so I will only share with you here, in a very summarized fashion, a few of the most powerful tools that I have found for balancing my hormones. I encourage you to do further research on this topic on your own if you suspect hormone imbalances are a contributing factor to your insomnia.

How to Discover Whether Your Hormones Need Help

For an excellent in-depth look at adrenal health, I recommend Dr. Lam's book, *Adrenal Fatigue: - Reclaim Your Energy and Vitality with Clinically Proven Natural Programs.* For great information on balancing the thyroid, I recommend either Janie Bowthorpe's book, *Stop the Thyroid Madness: A Patient Revolution Against Decades of Inferior Treatment*, and *Why Do I Still Have Thyroid Symptoms? When My Lab Tests Are Normal: a Revolutionary Breakthrough in Understanding Hashimoto's Disease and Hypothyroidism*, by Datis Kharrazian, DHSc, DC, MS.

If you are wondering whether an adrenal and/or thyroid disorder is causing you to get less than optimal rest, I recommend first asking your doctor to do a urine, blood and/or saliva test to measure your adrenal and thyroid hormones. If you don't have a good holistic integrative or naturopathic doctor, you'll want to find one, as most conventional medical doctors don't really understand how to balance the hormones. To find a good integrative and/or holistic doctor, I recommend consulting integrative medical associations such as the Academy for Comprehensive Integrative Medicine (ACIM), the American College for Advancement in Medicine (ACAM), or The Institute for Functional Medicine. For more information, see: ACIMConnect.com, ACAM.org and/or FunctionalMedicine.org. Consulting online support groups for referrals can also sometimes be beneficial.

Hormone balancing isn't a do-it-yourself endeavor though, so it's important to work with someone who can interpret test results for you and provide appropriate guidance about what you'll need. For your thyroid test, you'll want to do a complete blood panel that measures TSH, T4, T3, Free T3, T3 uptake, Hashimoto's antibodies and perhaps even Reverse T3.

For more information on what each of these tests measures, I recommend checking out the website: StopTheThyroidMadness.com. Alternatively, read Janie Bowthorpe's book, *Stop the Thyroid Madness: A Patient Revolution Against Decades of Inferior Treatment.* I also discuss some tips for addressing adrenal and thyroid dysfunction, especially in people with Lyme disease, in my 2012 book: *Beyond Lyme Disease: Healing the Underlying Causes of Chronic Illness in People with Borreliosis and Co-Infections.* To learn more, see: ConnieStrasheim.org/lyme-disease.

To measure your adrenal function, most holistic health care practitioners recommend doing a 24-hour saliva cortisol test. This should be combined with a clinical evaluation of your symptoms, since all tests have their limitations and none reveals perfectly what's going on in the body. I have known people to have near normal cortisol levels on a saliva test and yet have terrible adrenal fatigue, so it's important to work with a doctor who understands endocrine disorders (which, ironically, is not always a traditional endocrinologist but usually an integrative medical doctor or naturopath). Such doctors are usually able to diagnose you based on your symptoms, not just your test results.

A few of the most common symptoms of adrenal fatigue include:

- Morning fatigue
- Post-exertion malaise (which means that you become excessively tired or have an increase in symptoms as a result of doing too much)
- Low blood pressure
- Hypoglycemia
- Depression
- Anxiety
- Brain fog
- Gastrointestinal disturbances
- Insomnia
- Weight gain or weight loss

Hypothyroidism, which is the most common thyroid disorder, also causes depression, brain fog, fatigue and insomnia (among other symptoms) but for different reasons. Unfortunately, many people today battle both adrenal fatigue and thyroid dysfunction, especially those with autoimmune-like illnesses.

Tools for Restoring Optimal Adrenal Function

The most crucial step for restoring your adrenal glands, which is also the most difficult, yet the least expensive, is to cut down on the stress in your life! If you notice that you are constantly in "fight-or-flight" mode, rushing around, living in fear, taking on too many obligations, maintaining unhealthy relationships or working a stressful job—you must do what you can do reduce that stress. I realize that's really hard if you are living with heavy or multiple challenges, such as a chronic illness, financial hardship, or an abusive relationship—but the truth is, we can all do things to manage our response to challenging situations. This is the foremost step for recovery from this condition. Dr. Lam's book provides some excellent suggestions on how to do this.

Next, eliminate all inflammatory foods from your diet, as these foods stress the adrenal glands and cause them to overproduce cortisol, one of your body's principal stress hormones, which, when produced in excess, can keep you awake at night. Common inflammatory foods include: most dairy products, soy, wheat, gluten-containing foods, sugar, and of course, all foods that are excessively processed and which contain artificial ingredients (read: things that you can't grow or find in nature!).

One quick and easy guide on healthy eating is Michael Pollen's *Food Rules: An Eater's Manual.* This short book provides some easy-to-follow, simple guidelines for identifying healthy foods in the supermarket and is based more on concepts rather than a fixed dietary protocol. For information on how to tailor a diet to your specific needs, I recommend W. Lee Cowden, MDs and my 2014 book, *Foods that Fit a Unique You.* For more information, see: http://conniestrasheim.org/store/foods-that-fit-a-unique-you.

Third, ask your doctor about nutrients and supplements that support adrenal and thyroid function. Some of my favorites that promote adrenal health and which I have found to be safe for most people, include:

• Vitamin C (anywhere from 1,000 -30,000 mg daily, depending on your body's need. Start by taking 1,000 mg per day and add 500 mg daily to bowel tolerance. When your stools become slightly loose, reduce the dose slightly to get your optimal dose. At times during my recovery from Lyme disease, I have needed up to 20 grams (or 20,000 mg) daily of Vitamin C, so don't be surprised if you end up needing more than you think!

- Pantothenic acid or pantethine, also known as Vitamin B5. The adrenal glands love this nutrient. If you have adrenal fatigue, you'll want to include 500 mg or more as part of your daily regimen.

- Rhodiola or ashwagandha. These herbs are adaptogens that help to balance the adrenal hormones and many people seem to be able to tolerate them well.

- Licorice root or licorice root tea. Licorice is an excellent remedy if your cortisol levels are too low, since licorice causes your body to retain cortisol so that it stays in your body longer. Long- term use of licorice may cause hypokalemia or potassium depletion, so you'll want to monitor your potassium levels if you take licorice root long-term. Licorice root also boots the blood pressure, which is a great benefit for those of you who have low blood pressure (which is common in adrenal fatigue). However, it should be used only under physician supervision if you have heart disease, high blood pressure and/or high cortisol levels.

If you have advanced adrenal fatigue, which is characterized by profound fatigue, especially in the morning; anxiety, depression, an inability to exercise, weight fluctuations, gastrointestinal disturbances and low morning cortisol levels, or inverted or low cortisol levels across the board on a saliva test, you may also need to take bio-identical hormones and/or adrenal glandular formulas to balance your adrenal hormones. Bio-identical hormones compensate for whatever hormones your adrenal glands may not be making in sufficient amounts, and should be prescribed by a doctor who is an expert in bio-identical hormone supplementation.

Supplemental bio-identical hormones, like pregnenolone, progesterone, DHEA, 7-keto DHEA, testosterone and (as a last resort) hydrocortisone are all commonly prescribed to people with adrenal fatigue. These hormones provide powerful support to the adrenal glands and can help them to recover, while providing your body with the supplemental hormones that it needs.   The particular hormones that you'll need will depend upon your lab test results and symptoms.

Some of these hormones are more powerful than others, and have profound effects upon the body, so again, you'll want to work with a doctor who thoroughly understands bio-identical hormone replacement when deciding upon which one(s) would be most beneficial for you. It is beyond the scope of this book to describe the function of each of these hormones, so you'll want to do further research on your own to learn about how each of these hormones (among others) support the body.

Adrenal glandular formulas, such as those made by Standard Process and Biotics Research (such as Adrenal Dessicated and ADB5 Plus, respectively) contain bovine adrenal gland tissue and other nutrients, and are two glandular formulas that are widely recommended by many holistic and integrative doctors to support healthy adrenal function. Ideally, these should be used under physician supervision as well, since their effects upon the body can be profound and not everyone will respond well to them.

For more information on these products, see: StandardProcess.com and BioticsResearch.com.

Tools for Restoring Thyroid Function

If your thyroid dysfunction is mild or moderate, you may find that supporting your thyroid with thyroid hormone precursors such as iodine, selenium and L-tyrosine, or thyroid glandular formulas will restore your thyroid function back to normal. However, you'll want to work with your doctor to determine the specific products and dosages that you'll need.

Alternatively, and if your thyroid dysfunction is more severe as indicated by your symptoms and thyroid test results, you may benefit from taking bio-identical thyroid hormone medication. If you have adrenal fatigue along with thyroid dysfunction, you may respond better to a prescription of pure bio-identical T3 hormone, which is the active form of thyroid hormone that your body uses— rather than a combination of T4/T3. This is because in people with adrenal fatigue, the body will sometimes make Reverse T3 from T4 hormone (which is an inactive form of thyroid hormone) instead of the active T3 hormone that the body needs, and which can counteract the effects of T3.

To learn more about the interaction between adrenal and thyroid hormones, I recommend Dr. Lam's book, *Adrenal Fatigue - Reclaim Your Energy and Vitality with Clinically Proven Natural Programs* as well as Janie Bowthorpe's book, *Stop the Thyroid Madness*.

How Adrenal and Thyroid Disorders Disrupt Sleep

You may be wondering at this point how adrenal and thyroid disorders affect sleep. The mechanisms are multiple. First, the adrenals play a role in regulating inflammation, but when the body's cortisol levels are either too high or too low due to adrenal dysfunction, this leads to chronic inflammation, which causes sleep disturbances.

In addition, in adrenal dysfunction, the body's 24-cortisol rhythm is often thrown out of whack, and many people end up having too high levels of cortisol at night, which results in wakefulness and energy at night, and fatigue and sleepiness during the day.

Adrenal dysfunction can also cause hypoglycemia, resulting in the need to eat frequently. If you have hypoglycemia, you may tend to awaken in the middle of the night or early in the morning as your body releases adrenaline to mobilize glycogen reserves from your liver to increase your blood sugar. This too, will disrupt your sleep or keep you from getting a full night's rest.

Eating a protein or combination protein/fat snack before bedtime can help to stabilize your blood sugar throughout the night. And if you're like me, you'll find that a handful of nuts or a vegan protein shake just doesn't cut it. When my energy reserves are really depleted, I need a chicken leg or some bacon before bed! My friends make fun of me for eating at night, but I know that if I don't have some animal protein before bedtime, I'll awaken with hypoglycemia at 5 AM.

I constantly read in the media about how eating before bedtime is a bad idea. And at times, I have had doctors advise me to not eat within three hours of bedtime because nighttime is for detoxifying the body, not digestion. As true as this may be, I have found that every time that I have followed this advice, I have not been able to sleep as long or as deeply.

If you have hypoglycemic episodes during the night or awaken with adrenaline surging through your body (as indicated by a racing heart and/or feelings of shakiness or "buzzing"), you must eat before bedtime. If you don't, you can further destabilize your adrenal glands, which will lead to a cascade of other problems in your body, including even more compromised digestion and detoxification (the very reason some health experts believe you need to *not* eat before bedtime), and of course, insomnia.

If your test results show that your cortisol levels are high at night, ask your doctor about taking phosphatidylserine, which is a nutrient and phospholipid that lowers cortisol.

Thyroid dysfunction doesn't usually directly cause insomnia; it is often a byproduct of adrenal dysfunction though, and is important to treat along with the adrenal dysfunction in order for the whole endocrine system to work better.

How Hormonal Changes After 35 Keep You Awake at Night

If you are a pre-menopausal or menopausal woman, you may find that your sleep has become less than ideal, or even downright awful in recent years. Indeed, many women, sometime between the ages of 35-40, start experiencing sleep difficulties a few days or a week before their menstrual cycles, or throughout the month, as the hormones estrogen and progesterone start to become imbalanced as a natural result of aging. This results in insomnia. In women who are menopausal, these imbalances are often even greater.

Many women in midlife also have an imbalance of progesterone and estrogen partly because many environmental toxins act like estrogens in the body, and cause a condition called estrogen dominance. Phthalates, which are chemicals that are found in plastics, are a type of toxin that elevates estrogen in the body, and we are all filled with these chemicals. These xenoestrogens, or "fake estrogens" throw the body's natural balance of estrogen and progesterone off, resulting in low progesterone and artificially elevated levels of estrogen, which then causes insomnia and other symptoms.

Using a transdermal progesterone crème, which is available in most health food stores and online, can help to balance the ratio of progesterone to estrogen in your body and mitigate insomnia caused by too low levels of progesterone. Like all hormone replacement therapy, you shouldn't just take progesterone willy-nilly though, as it has profound effects upon the body, for better or for worse. Do a lab test to determine whether you need this, or any other hormone.

In addition, some supplements can help to remove or block the production of unwanted xenoestrogens in the body. DIM, or di-indolylmethane, may be one of the most famous of these. Certain foods such as flax seeds and sprouts, and cruciferous vegetables such as broccoli and cauliflower and cabbage are rich in indole-3-carbinol (I3C), a compound that the body converts to diindolylmethane (DIM).

According to gynecologist Christiane Northrup MD, author of *Women's Bodies, Women's Wisdom,* high estrogen levels are also associated with deficiencies of the vitamin B complex, especially vitamins B6 and B12, as well as vitamins C and E, magnesium and selenium. The liver requires adequate amounts of these nutrients to break down and inactivate estrogen, so you may want to also consider supplementing your diet with these vitamins and minerals, if you are a woman with PMS or menopausal symptoms that include insomnia and/or testing indicates that you need them.

Dr. Northrup's book provides additional excellent suggestions for reducing symptoms of PMS and menopause, including insomnia, and I highly recommend it for more information on this topic.

Low testosterone can also negatively affect sleep quality by disrupting deep sleep. It's not uncommon for women and men over 35 to have testosterone deficiencies, which is another good reason to get your hormones tested. If you are under 35, your hormonal imbalances may be less severe, unless you are battling a chronic illness, in which case you may also need bio-identical hormone replacement therapy, or supplemental nutrition to balance your hormones.

I began taking bio-identical hormones in the form of transdermal crèmes around age 37. My repertoire included pregnenolone, 7-keto DHEA and progesterone. My doctor prescribed these to me because I wasn't producing a sufficient amount of hormones due to Lyme disease and other stressors. When I began taking these hormones, my energy, mood and mental function all improved profoundly, along with my sleep.

I actually wish I had started taking bio-identical hormones sooner, since my hormone levels had been low for years and I was exhausted, brain fogged, depressed and continually sleep-deprived. I also discovered in my late 30s that my cholesterol levels were extremely low. The body creates all hormones from cholesterol, so this meant that my body didn't have enough raw material to make all the hormones that I needed in the first place. And if you don't have the raw material, or building blocks to make hormones, then that's a problem!

If you are battling a chronic health condition, you may want to get your cholesterol levels tested. If you have low healthy cholesterol, also called HDL cholesterol, you'll want to find ways to increase your levels of this crucial lipid (or fat). Cholesterol testing is a simple blood test that you can do through labs such as Quest or Lab Corp.

If you find that you are deficient in cholesterol, consider increasing your consumption of eggs and butter—two cholesterol-rich foods, and/or taking supplemental cholesterol, which you can purchase from the company New Beginnings at: nbnus.net. (Note: You'll need a doctor's note and lab test results to prove that you have low cholesterol, in order to purchase cholesterol from New Beginnings, which is, to my knowledge, the only company that makes it).

About Bio-Identical Hormone Replacement Therapy

Bio-identical hormone replacement therapy isn't for everyone, and hormone imbalances may or may not be the reason that you aren't getting enough shut-eye, so you'll want to get tested to find out for sure. Personally, taking supplemental hormones has been one of the most powerful things that I've ever done to regain my energy, stamina, mental clarity, and ability to sleep.

All of the hormones that I just described tend to be energizing, so if your doctor recommends them for you, you'll want to take them in the morning (except for progesterone, which is often sedating and should be used at night). Consider starting out on low doses and slowly increasing them over time, as if you take too much, too soon, or take hormones too late in the day, they can keep you awake at night.

In the long run, however, even energizing hormones can help you to sleep because they help to stabilize your adrenal glands and balance your overall chemistry. Again, hormone replacement is not a do-it-yourself project though, so I recommend working with a skilled practitioner in this area.

In summary, sleep is powerfully influenced by hormonal balance. Adrenal fatigue, hypothyroidism and other thyroid conditions, as well as hormonal changes around peri-menopause and menopause (in women) are some of the most common hormonal causes of insomnia. Imbalances can affect both your ability to fall asleep and stay asleep, so I recommend getting your hormones tested, especially if you are a woman over age 35 or are battling a chronic illness.

I believe that you'll be excited once you see the tremendous benefits that result when you balance your hormones with the proper nutrients, bio-identical hormones and a healthy diet. Indeed, addressing this aspect of your health can go a long way toward improving your quality of life, including your sleep.

Supporting my adrenal glands and thyroid with nutrition and bio-identical hormone replacement was only one piece of the sleep puzzle for me, but it was one of the most important.

As a final note, hormone replacement therapy is fantastic because it can also improve your emotional health, since adrenal dysfunction, thyroid hormone imbalances and female hormonal changes can all cause depression and anxiety, which have been linked to insomnia in many studies. By balancing your hormones, you are also balancing your mood, and along with that, your sleep.

Chapter Seven

Rest Better by Removing Pain and Chronic Infections

It is beyond the scope of this book to describe every possible cause of insomnia, but I want to briefly share a few solutions for two more major causes of insomnia, which you may not have thought of.

The first is physical pain. Many of us are awakened by pain, or simply can't fall asleep because of it. Throughout my journey with Lyme disease, I battled severe pain, especially muscle and joint pain in my lower back and right hip, which kept me tossing and turning many nights. To this day, I can only sleep on one side because lying on my stomach, back or left side causes the pain to return, but because I have a good system in place for managing the pain now, it no longer affects my sleep most of the time.

Create a Comfy Sleep Environment

I was able to significantly reduce the pain that I endured during every night by doing a few things. First, I invested in a supportive Tempurpedic mattress. When purchased new, these mattresses can cost $2,700 or more, but I found a slightly used one on Craigslist in excellent condition for around $1,200. I found the Tempurpedic bed to be the most supportive for my needs. In addition, I purchased a Mediflow water pillow, which I could fill with water according to the amount of support that I needed for my head and neck. For more information on these pillows, see: www.Mediflow.com.

You may find that you need a different type of bed; regardless, sleeping in a comfortable bed is important. This may sound like an obvious piece of advice, but I mention it because for years, I had thought that I was sleeping in a comfortable bed and that my back pain was all due to Lyme disease. I didn't realize until I bought a Tempurpedic bed how much better I could have been sleeping. It's an obvious thing that's not always so obvious!

Again, not everyone will do well with a Tempurpedic bed. For one thing, and like many mattresses, they are treated with chemicals that can cause an allergic reaction in some people. Because I bought mine slightly used and it had been in storage for a couple of years, I didn't have a problem with the mattress outgassing formaldehyde or other dangerous petrochemicals. These chemicals are often found in high levels in new mattresses, but some people may not be able to tolerate even used ones. Still, the Tempurpedic may be a good choice for some of you.

If you have chemical sensitivities, you may prefer to sleep on a mattress that is made of all natural materials and which hasn't been treated with dangerous chemicals. Dietrich Klinghardt, MD, PhD, in my 2016 book *New Paradigms in Lyme Disease Treatment: 10 Top Doctors Reveal Healing Strategies that Work,* recommends SAMINA mattresses, which have a grounding pad woven into them, and a climate-regulating wool pad topper. For more information, see:
http://justhealthysleep.com/sleeping-systems/.

There are other, less expensive options out there as well, which are made from materials such as organic cotton, wool and latex. Take your time to find a bed that works well for you. Some companies have a 30-day return policy on mattresses, which can be helpful when you are trying to find one that will give you deep, pain-free sleep.

Beds may be a costly investment for some of you, but a lack of sleep is also costly. If your mattress causes your back, neck or other parts of you to ache, and your funds are limited, I encourage you to look around your town or city for a slightly used or factory-returned mattress that alleviates your pain (if your pain is affected by the type of bed that you sleep on). Trust me, it will make a huge difference in the quality of your rest.

For years, I slept on only moderately supportive mattresses, not realizing that the pain that they caused were part of why I wasn't sleeping well and felt so miserable during the day. When I finally convinced myself that my health and sleep were worth investing in, I came up with a way to afford a better mattress.

Non-Toxic Pain Remedies

To further alleviate my pain, I used a variety of menthol and cannabis-based ointments on my lower hip and back, both of which are great for lowering inflammation. Sombra is one brand of menthol-based ointment that I like, because it is super effective and doesn't contain a lot of toxic chemical additives, unlike more conventional pain ointments sold in drugstores and pharmacies. It is also inexpensive and you can order it online; on Amazon and elsewhere. For more information on the products, see: http://www.sombrausa.com/.

Another great product that I have used for muscle, joint and nerve pain is a cannabis-based ointment from Mary's Medicinals: www.MarysMedicinals.com, which I purchased in Colorado, where you can get cannabis at dispensaries without a prescription. It contains just a tiny amount of THC (or tetrahydrocannabinol, the ingredient in cannabis that has psychotropic effects upon the mind). The THC in the product makes the cannabinoids work more effectively in the body, but it is not enough to affect mental function.

Indeed, I've found that cannabis pain and sleep products that contain just a small amount of THC are more effective than those that are made up of 100% cannabinoids, such as cannabinol (CBN) and/or CBD (cannabidoil), and which you can get just about anywhere, through reputable online companies such as Bluebird Botanicals. Still, products that contain 100% cannabinoids may be a viable option for those of you who live in states where cannabis products that contain THC are not yet legal. I have not found them to be as powerful or effective as those products that contain a little THC, but the 100% cannabinoid products may work well for you. For more information on CBD products from Bluebird Botanicals, see: www.bluebird-botanicals.com for more information.

Mary's Medicinals also sells transdermal pain patches, gel pens, CBD tinctures, capsules and other products. For more information, visit the Mary's Medicinals site: http://www.marysmedicinals.com/products-properties/.

Cannabis is an incredibly powerful tool for pain, as well as for sleep. (In the following section, I discuss its use as a sleep aid). It is so powerful in fact, that many people with a wide variety of health conditions, especially neurological diseases and cancer, have recently moved to states such as Washington and Colorado, where even recreational cannabis use is legal—just to be able to have access to this valuable plant. Fortunately, some other states are working to make cannabis use legal for medicinal purposes, so with any luck, we may all have access to it soon.

A couple of other products that I have found to work well for relieving pain and inflammation are DMSO and Tiger Balm. Tiger Balm is another menthol-based product, but it contains toxic chemicals, so I only recommend it as a last resort. Both products can be purchased at many online retailers.

If your pain is systemic and caused by infection, toxicity or hormonal imbalances, consider asking your doctor about a prescription for low-dose Naltrexone, which works on opioid receptors in the body and has been very effective for reducing pain and improving sleep in some people, especially those with neurological and other chronic disease conditions.

Finally, I have found Epsom salt baths, ice and heat packs and using a Biomat, which is an infrared mat that you lie on and which heats up—to all be effective for relieving pain of all kinds. Epsom salt baths and the Biomat are described later in this book.

Chronic Infections Cause Insomnia

Infections can be a major cause of insomnia. For instance, Lyme disease, which is a complex of multiple bacterial, parasitic and viral infections, often causes insomnia, particularly the protozoal infection *Babesia* and the bacterial infection *Bartonella*.

I don't fully understand all of the correlations between insomnia and infections, but many infections, such as those involved in Lyme disease, inflame the brain and neurological system, disrupt hormonal function and cause imbalances in many of the chemicals involved in sleep, especially the neurotransmitters. They also affect the health of the gastrointestinal tract, where many neurotransmitters are made.

In addition, in neurotoxic syndromes like Lyme disease, the body can become overloaded by toxins generated by the pathogens, as well as by toxins from the environment. Then, when the organs of elimination, such as the liver, gallbladder, lungs and kidneys, become overloaded trying to process these toxins, this can result in sleeplessness.

If you are battling chronic infections, the involved pathogens or the problems that they cause in your body may be hindering your ability to sleep.

The obvious first step to resolving insomnia caused by infections is to treat the infections. It is beyond the scope of this book to describe how to do that, but I highly recommend consulting with a reputable integrative or naturopathic doctor, or other qualified health care practitioner who uses outside-the-box methods for detecting and treating infections, in addition to conventional lab tests. This is because most conventional lab tests cannot detect many chronic infections, such as those caused by Lyme disease.

Sophisticated lab testing and tools such as Autonomic Response Testing (ART) and other forms of bio-energetic testing are often more reliable than conventional labs for detecting the chronic, stealth infections that many of us have. For more information on energetic testing, see Dr. Cowden's and my book, *BioEnergetic Tools for Wellness*.

You may also find that removing the toxins from your body using a variety of detoxification therapies can help you to sleep. Coffee enemas, castor oil packs over the liver, body brushing, rebounding, sauna therapy and taking homeopathic detoxification remedies such as those by Pekana and NutraMedix, are a few of the tools that doctors recommend to facilitate toxin removal through the liver, gallbladder, kidneys, skin and lymphatic system. For more information on how to detoxify your body, you may want to read Dr. Cowden's and my short book *Create a Toxin-Free Body or Home...Starting Today*.

Finally, even if you are battling infections and an overload of toxins, all of the sleep tools that I mention in this book are still likely to help you. You don't have to remove every last trace of infection in your body before these tools will be effective for you. That said, the more that you are able to eliminate the infections and toxins from your body, the fewer tools you may need in the long run to sleep at night.

Chapter Eight

Relax Your Body and Mind with Cannabis and Botanical and Homeopathic Remedies

Cannabis for Sleep

I highly recommend low-THC, high CBD/CBN cannabis formulas for sleep, in addition to pain. Interestingly, cannabinol (or CBN), which is an aged cannabinoid, or compound found in cannabis, is more effective than CBD for improving sleep. The Indica strains of cannabis (and CBN) in particular, are very calming to the nervous system, and very effective for relieving pain, anxiety and insomnia. A handful of studies substantiate this. For instance, one study, the results of which were published in the journal *Neurology* on September 27, 2005, showed that cannabis was helpful for reducing pain and sleep disturbances in patients with multiple sclerosis related central neuropathic pain, and was mostly well tolerated.[viii]

Cannabis has been given a bad rap by the media, but most studies have shown cannabis to be non-toxic to the body. And the good news is, you don't have to "get high" to enjoy the benefits of cannabis for sleep. Many Indica strains of cannabis contain very little THC (again, that compound that has psychotropic effects upon the mind) and are very relaxing and healing to the nervous system. THC has its own health benefits, but it's not for everyone and you don't really need it for sleep, since it's the compounds in the plant called cannabinoids (especially CBN) that generally induce relaxation and sleep.

Like all medicines, cannabis can be abused, and the high-THC products are not appropriate for everyone, due to their mind and mood-altering effects. However, the cannabinoids in low THC products are generally very safe and well-tolerated by many people, and overall, cannabis has been shown to have fewer side effects than most over-the -counter drugs like Advil PM and Benadryl (both of which have been shown in studies to cause Alzheimer's dementia with prolonged use).

Mary's Medicinals makes some wonderful products for sleep; I have found their CBN capsules and creams to work well for this purpose. The capsules contain 5 mg of cannabinol per capsule and just a tiny amount of THC. Effective doses depend upon the person, but I have found that I can safely take 2 capsules at a time. You may find that you need a bit more, or even less (say, half a capsule). For more information, see: MarysMedicinals.com.

Cannabis is also available in many other forms; as a tincture, vaporized, in food products, etc. but I find that the capsules are the easiest and simplest way to take it for a peaceful night's rest. You can experiment with different forms to find one that works well for you.

The Biomat: A Great Relaxant and Pain-Reducer

Another great pain-relieving and sleep-inducing tool that I recommend is the Biomat, which is a therapeutic mat that you lie on and which heats up your body. It contains far infrared rays, negative ions and amethyst crystals, all of which deliver relaxing, regenerative and deep-penetrating heat to your tissues. It is a fantastic tool for those of you who struggle to fall asleep at night due to pain or a simple inability to wind down.

The technology of the Biomat is based on Nobel prize-winning scientific research pioneered by NASA and is effective for helping to heal the body of a variety of conditions, including insomnia and pain. Among the other benefits of the Biomat, and according to the Biomat site, this therapeutic mat also "repairs damaged tissue, reduces joint and muscle soreness, chronic neck and back pain, toxicity, oxidation levels, inflammation and arthritis, and circulatory issues."

I recommend checking out the Biomat as an additional option for resolving both pain and insomnia, and for maintaining overall wellness. Biomats range from $600 (for a mini-biomat) to $1900 for a full-sized mat.
  For more information, check out the website:
www.BioMat.com.

Magnesium Sulfate: A Cheap Relaxant

Another inexpensive pain-reducing tool that also induces relaxation is a hot Epsom salt bath, taken right before bedtime. Epsom salts contain magnesium sulfate, which relax the muscles and draw inflammation-causing toxins out of the tissues. If your sleep issues are severe, a bath isn't likely to be enough to get you to sleep, but Epsom salt baths can help you to unwind at night and at times, take the edge off of your pain.

Sleep-Inducing Botanical Remedies

Many of the botanical remedies that are commonly prescribed for sleep, such as passionflower, chamomile, kava kava and valerian, as well as popular essential oils like lavender, can be helpful for sleep. However, I've found that for many people that I know who have severe neurological illnesses they generally aren't as effective or powerful as some of the other tools that I describe here. I have tried many of them over the years, and frankly, they didn't do whole lot to resolve my insomnia. This is probably because many factors were contributing to the dysfunction in my body, and I had to address those with tools that were specific to the problems that I had. You'll want to do the same.

However, I believe that botanical remedies can and do work for many people, which is why I mention them here. They just weren't enough for me. Many of the calming herbal remedies and essential oils are great simply because they are generally non-toxic, gentle and inexpensive. Some of the more popular botanicals include:

- Valerian
- Skullcap
- Jamaican dogwood
- Chamomile
- Passionflower
- Lavender
- Kava kava

You can find these online or at your local health food store. As with all supplements, you'll want to use a product that has been recommended by a qualified health care professional and which has a solid track record of effectiveness.

Sleep-Inducing Homeopathic Remedies

While I did not use homeopathic remedies as part of my sleep toolbox, they too, can be effective for restoring sleep, if they are prescribed according to the specific condition for which you need them. Following is an excerpt on homeopathic remedies, taken from Dr. Cowden's and my 2014 book, *BioEnergetic Tools for Wellness*.

Reprinted from BioEnergetic Tools for Wellness, copyright 2014, by William Lee Cowden, MD and Connie Strasheim

We recommend homeopathic and energetic remedies for sleep because they are gentle and inexpensive, and at times, can be targeted, or tailored, to the specific cause of your insomnia. We recommend that you choose a homeopathic remedy based on the characteristics and type of insomnia that you have, as well as your personal constitution and history. There are a wide variety of remedies to choose from, and you may find it most useful to work with a homeopath or other holistic doctor experienced in their use, to determine the one(s) that would best fit you.

You can get insights into the remedy or remedies that are most adequate for you and your particular situation by reading homeopath David Curtin's article, "Sleep Problems" featured on the British Homeopathic Association webpage: BritishHomeopathic.org.

This page contains a list of some commonly used remedies for insomnia and for what circumstances each remedy is indicated. For instance, Nux vomica is a remedy that is useful for people who awaken around 3 a.m., with their brain full of thoughts. Coffee is useful when you are completely sleepless, or if you sleep until 3 a.m. but then are awake or doze the rest of the night. Belladonna is helpful if you have anxious, frightful or vivid dreams. Other remedies described on the webpage include: stramonium, valeriana, pulsatilla and arsenicum, among others.

Homeopathic remedies are generally safe and non-toxic, so if your time or finances are limited, you could try using one or more of these remedies on your own, before consulting with a healthcare practitioner. If that doesn't prove to be an effective strategy, you might then consider working with an experienced homeopath to see if you get better results.

Some other energetically imprinted herbal remedies for sleep include the NutraMedix products Babuna and Amantilla (NutraMedix.com), which are energetically imprinted chamomile and valerian root extracts, respectively. According to Dr. Cowden, Babuna may be especially effective for children, and Amantilla for adults. For more information on these remedies, see: NutraMedix.com.

The Benefits of Melatonin

No sleep book would be complete without including a discussion of melatonin, which is the hormone that the pineal gland in your brain naturally produces at night to help you fall asleep and stay asleep. Many of us don't produce enough melatonin nowadays, due to disrupted or inverted sleep-wake cycles, toxins, illness, hormonal dysfunction due to stress, and other factors. Using computers and exposing yourself to bright light late at night can also disrupt your body's production of melatonin, since melatonin is produced in conditions of complete darkness.

To optimize your body's melatonin production, avoid bright light late at night or within two hours of bedtime, and get as much sunlight as you can during the day. Sunlight causes your body to produce serotonin, which converts to melatonin at night.

You can also take supplemental melatonin, which is available at health food stores and online. While some health care practitioners don't recommend taking melatonin on a long-term basis, I have found that many people who have battled severe chronic illness need to do so, and other practitioners feel that this is okay. So the issue is a bit controversial, but I've found long-term melatonin supplementation to be necessary for some people, myself included.

Melatonin doses range from .5 mg per night up to 10 mg per night. It's one of those things that some people need just a little bit of, while others need a lot of. Paradoxically, it can worsen insomnia if you take too much. For instance, I found that my ideal dose for years was 1.5 milligrams, 30 minutes before bedtime. If I took more than that, I had vivid nightmares and did not sleep deeply. As I entered my 40s, I found that I needed a bit more, so I've since then increased my dose to 2.5 mg and found that to be more than adequate. You'll want to consult with your local healthcare practitioner to find a dose that works for you.

One side benefit of melatonin is that it is a free radical scavenger that protects the brain against the damaging effects of neurotoxins and as such, is also a powerful anti-cancer hormone. Indeed, through my interviews with integrative and holistic cancer doctors, I've found that many doctors use melatonin as an adjunct cancer treatment, in doses of 10 mg or more. However, I do not recommend taking such high doses except under physician supervision.

For the purpose of sleep, most people don't need more than that anyway, and as with all supplements, I recommend starting out on a lower dose; say 1 mg, and gradually increasing it from there, depending on your body's response.

Because melatonin is a hormone and the effects of long-term supplementation are relatively unknown, I don't recommend it as a first line of defense when treating insomnia. But, you may find that you need it, in addition to some of the other tools described in this book, if melatonin deficiency is causing your insomnia. It is, in any case, probably much safer than any sleep medication on the market.

Chapter Nine

Discover The King Method: a Free, Hands-On Healing Tool

About the King Method (TKM®)

Note: Excerpts from this section have been taken from BioEnergetic Tools for Wellness, © 2014 by Lee Cowden, MD and Connie Strasheim and modified to fit the context of this book.

The King Method (TKM®) is a simple, inexpensive hands-on healing technique that can help you to sleep by calming your nervous system and balancing your body's entire bio-electromagnetic system. It is a profoundly simple but powerful tool that I have found helps me to fall asleep when my nervous system is overactive. It also helps me to relax and return to sleep if I awaken in the middle of the night or in the early morning with my mind full of thoughts. The best news about this technique is that its foundational sequence, called the Median Sequence, is free and easy to learn, and you can do it from the comfort of your bed.

There are many hands-on sequences in TKM, each of which are used to treat a specific ailment or condition. The basic Median Sequence, which is the core sequence, is used to balance your body's energy, and takes just a few minutes to learn and about 20-40 minutes to do (depending on how much benefit you want to receive from it). It involves calming your body's energy field by lightly placing the pads of your fingers over certain locations on your body for 5-10 minutes per location.

TKM is based on the idea that the bio-electromagnetic system of your physical body governs its wellbeing, and that when this system works well, the body functions properly. Glenn King, PhD, CDN, CN, and Director of the King Institute, Inc., developed TKM after learning about the physics of the body's bio-electromagnetic system and how it affects human health. TKM is the product of Dr. King's discoveries, spiritual revelations from God, and the studies of others.

The cultural roots of TKM can be traced to the Orient and perhaps even to ancient Greece, although Dr. King credits God with ultimately teaching him how to develop the technique, since his revelations about TKM have resulted from extensive prayer, along with his studies and research.

According to the The King Institute website: "The King Institute Method® (TKM®) is an extraordinary hands-on approach to health disorders. This method has been shown to have a profound effect on the bio-electromagnetic systems of the body, which affect all bio-systems. The initial understanding of TKM® has been effectively utilized to treat people for years for common to complex disorders." So TKM isn't just useful for restoring sleep, but also for alleviating the symptoms of a multitude of health conditions.

According to Dr. King, TKM is not a renaming of any other kind of hands-on therapy, and is a unique method to naturally heal the body. Unlike some other types of hands-on therapy, it does not draw upon outside energies, only the body's innate electromagnetic energy.

Also, TKM energy pathways are different from the meridian energy pathways commonly described in bioenergetic medicine. According to Dr. King, there are different levels, or densities of energy in the human body, which precede one another. They are also interdependent, connecting with one another. TKM energy pathways go deeper than meridian energy, which is a more superficial level of energy circulation in the body.

The many sequences involved in TKM take a bit of practice and time to learn, but the basic Median sequence almost anyone can do, and it can be profoundly beneficial for helping some people to relax and fall asleep faster.

The King Institute boasts many healing testimonials on its website which demonstrate the effectiveness of TKM for treating a variety of acute and chronic conditions, including insomnia. Thousands of people, including many with medically incurable diseases or genetic disorders, have been healed by this unique hands-on therapy.

How to Do The Median Sequence (A Self-Help Sequence)

Sit or preferably lie in a comfortable position. For best results, remove all metallic objects from your body and clothing, including underwire bras, watches, belts and jewelry. It's best to wear 100 percent cotton clothing, and to position pillows beneath your arms, so that your muscles can completely relax as you apply each step of the procedure.

Next, go to the following link for complete and yet simple instructions on how to do the technique. This link also

contains an easy-to-follow diagram that illustrates the Median Sequence:
https://www.kinginstitute.org/attachments/article/319/M EDIAN%20Seq..pdf.

As you can see, for this sequence, you will simply be placing the pads (not the tips) of your first three fingers (index, middle, and ring), palm side down, on different points (areas) of your body, for a period of five minutes on each area. Or, if you wish, you may use all of your finger pads. You don't need to apply pressure to your skin with your fingers; in fact, this can inhibit the effectiveness of the process. Contacting your body (even through a single layer of clothing) is all that is needed to stimulate energy circulation.

Dr. King has developed other TKM sequences to help heal the body of a multitude of chronic and degenerative conditions. For more information on these sequences, visit: TheKingInstitute.org.

Chapter Ten

Practice Proper Sleep Hygiene with Healthy Nighttime Habits

Nearly every single book that I've read on sleep contains a section on proper sleep hygiene. I used to skip right over those sections because I didn't think that they would be helpful for me. In my frustrated, sleep-deprived state, I would think, *I have a neurological illness that keeps me awake, no matter how sleep-deprived I am or what I do, and somebody wants to tell me that going to bed at the same time every night and taking a hot bath is going to make some kind of difference?"*

As much as I felt like some of these authors didn't understand the challenges of those with complex neurological illnesses, over time, I let go of my pride as I realized how powerful proper sleep habits and sleep hygiene actually are—no matter the reason why you can't sleep in the first place. They can help to put you on the fast track to better rest, when they are combined with other sleep tools.

Part of proper sleep hygiene means learning to adopt healthy sleep habits (if you aren't doing that already). In the beginning, changing long-standing habits can be difficult, especially if you seem to have no circadian rhythm and don't fall asleep or get up at the same time—ever! Your body may initially refuse to cooperate with your intention to go to bed at the same time every night or get up at the same time every day, which means that it will be challenging at first to stick to a set sleep schedule.

Yet if you determine to get up at the same time every day and you set an alarm to do this, chances are, over time you will more readily fall asleep at the same time every night, and tend to get up at the same time in the morning. You may have to endure more sleep deprivation at first when you do this, but after a few weeks, your body should begin to adjust. Trust me though—I know how difficult this is. If you haven't slept for two nights in a row and then you sleep on the third night, you'll desperately want to sleep in late the next day because you now feel half-dead! It's okay; I promise it will get easier with time.

Exposing yourself to bright sunlight or using a sunlamp first thing in the morning for 20-30 minutes can make the process easier because it will help to change your body's circadian rhythm, or sleep-wake cycle, as will being as active as you can during the day and taking plenty of time to wind down before bedtime.

Another great strategy for cultivating an earlier, or more uniform, sleep-wake cycle is to get a sound-light machine, which I described earlier. This device can help you to fall asleep more quickly and easily. Use it right after you climb into bed so that you're asleep within 30-40 minutes of your target bedtime.

A brilliant pharmacist who specializes in sleep disorders once told me that it's more important to get up at the same time every day than go to bed at the same time every night (although aiming for a uniform sleep-wake cycle is optimal). So if you miss your scheduled bedtime by 30 minutes, or even an hour at first, it's apparently not as much of a big deal as getting up at a random time every day.

I have more energy at night and I do my best work at night, so the kid in me tends to kick and scream when it's time for bed. I'd rather stay up and work or read a good book. Trust me, that good book will do you in and keep you up later than you need to be! Find something relatively boring or relaxing to read instead so that you don't mind putting the book down after 15-20 minutes in bed.

When winding down or trying to adjust to a new set bedtime, consider taking a hot bath, lying on a Biomat, or listening to meditation CDs (more on these later) before bed to help you relax.

It's also essential to unplug any glowing gadgets in your room, and to get off of your computer and cellphone at least a couple of hours prior to bedtime. The light and electromagnetic frequencies from these devices stimulate the pineal gland in your brain, throw your energy balance off, and keep you awake much longer, or keep you from getting into the deeper stages of sleep.

I used to read my emails and peruse Facebook while in the bathtub right before bed. It was the only time of day that I could read my email and check out what was happening on social media, but just 20 minutes of Facebook or Internet time would often keep me awake for an hour or two past my scheduled bedtime.

In addition, the EMFs that cell phones radiate nowadays are extremely high (even when you are just texting or perusing the Internet), and are damaging to the brain and body, so using your phone to regularly consult Facebook, your email or the Internet really isn't a good idea. I interview cancer doctors for a living and a few have shared with me that they are seeing many more people with brain cancer today than they did 20 years ago—even in children. The reason is excessive cellphone use. What's more, the Internet, and especially social media like Facebook have become an addiction for many people, and while it's great to be better connected to the world, it can replace more meaningful face-to-face relationships and activities. Balance is key, I think.

If you are in a difficult battle with insomnia, you'll want to do calming activities for an hour or two before bedtime. Read an uplifting book, watch a lighthearted show on TV (news, violent shows and other negative media can actually create anxiety and prevent sleep), listen to some meditative CDs or calming music, sit in a sauna, pray, do some gentle stretches or take a hot bath. You want to head to bed in a peaceful, positive and relaxed frame of mind.

Finally, if you are like me, and your sleep-wake cycle has been wrecked by years of drugs, trauma and neurodegenerative disease, you may find that you need to sleep in a completely dark, cool, comfortable and quiet room to get deep, restful sleep. This can be tough to achieve if you are in a hotel or have lots of noisy neighbors, but I have found a few things to help with this process.

First, if you're traveling and know that the place where you'll be staying doesn't have thick curtains to darken the room, I recommend bringing some tinfoil or black fabric with you to drape over the windows. Tinfoil does a great job of blocking out bright light, and while not convenient to use, it works when you have nothing else around.

I use blackout curtains at home, and turn on a loud Austin Air purifier on High while I sleep so that I don't hear my neighbor upstairs clomping around at 6 AM. When I travel, I use high-decibel earplugs and request hotel rooms that are at the far end of the hallway, away from the elevator, pool, other rooms and street noise. It's a bit of a pain, but it's well worth it.

When I was in my 20s, before I got Lyme disease, I traveled overseas a lot and used to sleep in hostels that housed six people to a room, and somehow, I managed to get enough rest. But since contracting Lyme disease and suffering damage to my neurological system, I'm now only able to sleep in quiet hotels with supportive mattresses. It costs a lot more money to travel this way, but if I want to function on my trips, I have to do it.

So while I sleep relatively well at home, getting enough sleep when I travel or when I'm under a lot of stress, can occasionally still be a challenge for me. Fortunately, I've found cannabis to be a great alternative to benzodiazepine drugs when I need something extra to get by, and on those rare occasions when even the cannabis doesn't work (because, for example, I'm under a lot of stress, in an exceptionally noisy, hot room or uncomfortable bed), I will often take nothing additional to sleep and instead choose to suffer the effects of sleep deprivation.

I do this because I know that the alternative, which is to take a mind-altering, memory-erasing medication, is a slippery path that leads to life-destroying addiction down the road, no matter how often I might try to convince myself that I can take the pill "just this once." I tried that for years, thinking that if I just took benzos on occasion, whenever I traveled two or three times a year, that I would be okay.

It took a few hard relapses for me to realize that one pill would eventually lead to two pills, and then to three. According to UK addictions counselor, Baylissa Frederick, author of *Recovery and Renewal: Your Essential Guide to Overcoming Dependency and Withdrawal from Sleeping Pills, Other 'Benzo' Tranquillisers and Antidepressants*, in the UK, long-term use of sedatives is considered to be just two weeks! In other words, addiction can occur in that short amount of time for some people.

This meant that taking sedatives on a two-week trip was not okay for me. The final straw was when, after a number of years of intermittently taking benzodiazepines, I began to suffer severe withdrawal symptoms as a result of taking the drug *just once*. I then realized that I could never touch it again, as withdrawal effects tend to increase over time and the more you relapse.

If you are on sedative drugs, antidepressants or other medications prescribed for sleep, and decide to wean off of them, I encourage you to determine to never take them again, once you are off of them, no matter how much sleep you might miss out on. They will destroy your brain and the rest of your body. Just because they are legal and doctors prescribe them, does not mean they are safe. They are worse than many street drugs.

I realize that some of you who have severe chronic health issues may need to take them at times because the pain or insomnia you endure are just too great, and you are willing to endure the cost of taking them. I deeply empathize with you (no judgment, really!) but know that they carry a heavy price tag and you'll want to consider a better solution for the long term. For most problems, including insomnia, there are better alternatives. But again, if you decide to get off of sleep medication at some point, you'll want to work with a skilled healthcare practitioner who understands sleep medication addiction and how to safely withdraw from it.

Chapter Eleven

Heal from the Emotional and Spiritual Causes of Insomnia

Stress, Anxiety and Depression Underlie Sleep Disorders

Nearly all of us don't sleep at times due to stress. Perhaps you recall not being able to sleep before an important exam, or a big trip across the country, or after a fight with your significant other. Occasional sleeplessness isn't a big deal, but when you begin taking the worries of life to bed with you every night, that's a problem.

Stress, anxiety and depression often underlie sleep disorders, even if there is also a biochemical or environmental reason for the insomnia. The stress may even be subconscious or unconscious; for example, memories of trauma can be stored in the body, unbeknownst to the sufferer, who is awakened by night terrors or nightmares, or who can't fall asleep or stay asleep due to the trauma. The limbic system also tends to function on "high alert" in people with long-standing trauma, which can lead to frequent sleeplessness.

Fear of Not Sleeping Produces Sleeplessness

This is another problem. When you don't sleep well for months, or years, you begin to fear not being able to sleep. And if you are like I was, you know that the battle with insomnia can become so intense that at times, the lack of sleep and fear of not sleeping becomes traumatic, and worsens the insomnia.

If this is you, I get it. For years, I battled incredible fears about what might happen to me if I never slept well again. Often, I sobbed throughout the entire night, because I had spent years in the prison of insomnia and after many years of searching, I believed that there were no answers (or so I thought!) The chronic sleep deprivation, along with Lyme disease, messed with my thoughts and even caused me to believe at times that life wasn't worth living, as I wondered what I would do if I never had a good night of rest, ever again. Those of you who have endured this kind of thing know that I am not exaggerating in the slightest about how incredibly difficult this is to endure.

While trauma causes chronic insomnia, chronic insomnia is in itself traumatic and can breed more trauma; terrorists and militaries worldwide use insomnia as a form of torture on prisoners. When you don't sleep, day after day, month after month, and even year after year—life begins to look incredibly dismal, and all sorts of fears can take over your mind. If you were like me, at times you might fear never being able to sleep again, or that the lack of sleep is going to kill you. You then fear that there is nothing out there that will help you, and that there is no hope because your chemistry or emotions or whatever it happens to be—are just too messed up.

But I am here to tell you that it's not true. You are not beyond help or hope! It took me years to find my way back to getting a solid seven or eight hours of rest every night, and if I did it, then I truly believe that you can, too. I had many problems: a traumatic upbringing, a brain that had been damaged by Lyme disease and over ten years of chronic anti-depressant and benzodiazepine use; chronic fatigue, adrenal insufficiency, and living quarters that were less than ideal. Yet over time, I found solutions for most of these issues. There is nothing that you battle that can't be resolved!

Tools for Overcoming Fear and Worry

If you have begun to dread going to bed at night or aren't sleeping simply because you fear you won't sleep, the first thing that you'll need to do is find a strategy to overcome that fear.

Most fears that we have aren't based in reality or upon solid evidence, but if you have battled chronic insomnia for years, you know that your fear of not sleeping *is* based in reality. However, it isn't usually the fear of not sleeping that is the problem; it is the beliefs and catastrophic thinking that often go along with that fear, which then leads to other fears.

Thoughts such as "I'm going to feel horrible tomorrow if I don't sleep..." or, "I'll never be able to live as long as I don't sleep," or "What if I can't function? What if I can't attend work or a meeting, or go out with friends if I don't sleep tonight?" –Are common in those with chronic sleep deprivation and can cause great torment.

Breaking the "What if" and other catastrophic thinking patterns can be difficult. After all, your fears are based in a reality that has proven to be true, time and again. Sleep deprivation *does* make you feel horrible and *does* cause you to not be able to function. Perhaps it has even incapacitated you and made you sick.

It rarely works to just try to push catastrophic thoughts aside, especially when you find yourself tossing and turning for hours, it's 3 AM, and you've run out of options. You need to have more peaceful, relaxing and positive thoughts at the ready to replace the catastrophic ones. To do this, I have found all of the following strategies to be helpful:

- Writing down the lies or harmful beliefs that you have learned to embrace because of the insomnia, and asking God, a friend or a counselor to give you a positive truth to replace each one of those lies. This is so that when the lies surface at 2 AM, you have some powerful truths sitting at your bedside on a piece of paper that you can immediately grab and speak aloud, to counter the lies and fill your mind with.

  For instance, an example of one lie that you might believe is, "I will never sleep again and there is no way out." You could replace that thought with, "I haven't yet tried every sleep solution that's out there, and just because I haven't slept for X number of years doesn't mean that I won't ever sleep again. Many people have battled insomnia for years and yet found a way out. I will, too."

- Listening to guided relaxation or meditative CDs or MP3 downloads can help you to relax and take your focus off of your fears. For instance, you may be asked during a guided relaxation CD to visualize in detail a vacation spot, while soft, soothing instrumental plays in the background. I have found guided relaxation CDs to be useful when I have a lot on my mind, as well as when I fear not being able to sleep. One good resource for information on meditative and relaxation CDs is Insomnia.net: http://www.insomnia.net/natural-remedies/cds/.

- Giving your fears over to God and asking Him to do what you can't do, which is help you to sleep, and then consciously affirming aloud that you trust Him to do what you can't in your own power and strength. You let go of the outcome, trusting your Creator to provide what you need instead of trying to do it all yourself. You almost have to get to a place where you can say, "I don't care if I don't sleep. So what if the worst happens? So what if I die and go to the Afterlife? Would that be so bad?"

It has often been said that there is no worse fear than fear itself. So letting go of your life, in every sense of the word, not in resignation, but in surrender, allows the power of God to come in and do for you what you can't do for yourself. And I have found that God is real, good and trustworthy, and He is willing and able to help anyone who asks Him for help. Ask, and then trust that it will be done for you. You don't have to have all of the answers. You simply surrender it all, and as you do, you'll find yourself falling asleep more easily.

As part of my "letting go" process, I found it helpful to meditate on Scriptures in the Bible that spoke of God's love and care for me. I believe that there is supernatural power in the words of the Bible, and that by meditating upon these words and speaking them aloud, power is released into the atmosphere and this then changes things in the natural realm.

Of course, meditating upon and speaking any positive words can have a beneficial effect upon your mind and body. The important thing to know is this: your words have the power to create and change your circumstances, for better or for worse.

It can take time to learn how to replace catastrophic thinking with more beneficial, peaceful thoughts. Don't get discouraged if at first you don't sense any change or find the catastrophic thoughts taking over your mind again as soon as you stop your meditations. Over time, and the more that you practice replacing harmful thoughts with happy ones, this will change. Mental strongholds and negative thinking patterns take time to get ingrained into the mind, which means that they can take time to dislodge, too. But with persistence and by filling your mind as often as you can with positive thoughts, you will find your mental patterns changing.

Science has even proven that we can change the neural pathways in our brains when we practice positive thinking. This means that you can change your brain's chemistry by choosing peaceful, positive and empowering thoughts daily. I realize this can be *very* hard to do when you are sleep deprived, but every little change that you can make in the right direction will move you one step closer toward more restful sleep.

So don't give the insomnia more power than it already has by meditating upon it! You will dismantle its power over your life by ignoring it (again, I know this is hard when you feel awful and are terribly sleep-deprived) but when you choose to do or focus on other things, you diminish its hold upon your life.

- Remember that you have not tried every single sleep tool that is out there, and that just because you have endured insomnia for months or years, doesn't mean that there isn't a way out. One of the most difficult and tortuous thoughts that I had while weaning off of sleep medication was that there was no way out. I would even tell people, "I feel like there's no way out!"

During such times, I would ask God to speak His truths to me, which were inevitably that there *was* a way out for me, and that in time, He would show it to me. If you start to have thoughts like I did, just remember, you haven't tried everything, and even if you don't know what to do next, you can surrender it all and trust that an answer will be brought to you when you don't know where to find it.

As a side note, trusting in a loving God can be difficult if you haven't experienced Him or known Him to be good, or your image of Him reflects that of the authority figures in your life who perhaps didn't take care of you as well as they should have, or if others have beat you over the head with religion.

If this is you, I encourage you to ask God to reveal Himself to you, and to show you who He truly is, apart from what you've learned about Him from the authority figures and other people in your life. Ask Him to tell you the truth about who He is and the plan that He has for your life. Then, find a quiet place to retreat to, and listen, as He speaks to you. He will likely begin to orchestrate circumstances in your life to reveal Himself to you.

- Finally, some people have found it helpful to simply get up and do something when they can't sleep and/or fear not sleeping. Do some work, read a book, or just *something* until you are finally exhausted enough to fall asleep and the fear of not sleeping has been shoved to the back burner by your focusing on another activity. This strategy did not work well for me, but I know of others who have tried it and found it to be beneficial.

How to Heal from Trauma

Trauma, especially emotional trauma, can cause chronic insomnia, as memories of traumatic events remain lodged in the subconscious or unconscious mind and body and perpetually keep the nervous system in overdrive, or on high alert. Trauma, especially when prolonged, entrains the limbic system to operate largely in "fight or flight" mode or sympathetic overdrive. In this state, the body is continually flooded with stimulatory neurochemicals such as epinephrine and adrenaline, which can keep you awake at night.

Unfortunately, insomnia is also a natural outcome of post-traumatic stress disorder (PTSD), which is linked to trauma and can lead to nightmares or cause you to become afraid to fall asleep. People who have PTSD live on "high alert" as their brains get stuck in a pattern of constantly feeling threatened by danger, whether real or perceived, and this too can prevent them from falling asleep or sleeping deeply. People who have experienced ongoing trauma often awaken easily at the slightest noise, having learned to be hyper vigilant.

Some of you may even have experienced in-utero trauma while you were in your mother's womb. Your conscious mind does not remember this trauma, but it is lodged in your subconscious, or unconscious mind and body. Studies have shown that memories aren't just stored in the mind, but in the organs and tissues, as well.

Some people have found it very helpful do mind-body techniques to eliminate the trauma from the body as well as the mind, and to "reprogram" the limbic system. It is beyond the scope of this book to go into every mind-body tool that's out there, but a few great mind-body healing tools that I like and which you may want to investigate on your own include:

- Dynamic Neural Retraining System (DNRS). This program helps to de-program the limbic system out of a habitual "fight or flight" response and restore normal function to the brain and body. For more information visit the DNRS site: www.RetrainingtheBrain.com.

- The King Method (TKM). TKM is a manual, hands-on technique (described earlier) that balances your body's energy and as a byproduct sometimes releases emotions that are stored in the body.   For more information, see: www.KingInstitute.org.

- Inner healing prayer ministry. This involves inviting God into your memories and asking Him to supernaturally heal the underlying harmful beliefs and thought patterns that may have resulted from past experiences.

There are various forms of inner healing ministry, like Theophostic and Sozo ("sozo" in Greek means to save, deliver, protect, heal, preserve, do well, and be made whole), among many others. Unlike traditional counseling and some other emotional healing tools, inner healing prayer relies more upon the supernatural power of God to heal rather than upon the person receiving the healing. The person who receives the healing still participates to some degree, but it is God who supernaturally effectuates change in the mind and body.

There are a number of trained healing ministers who do inner healing work, but really good ones who are truly in tune with the Spirit of God can be difficult to find. Nonetheless, I believe that it is a very powerful way to be healed of past trauma, because the healing comes about as a result of a supernatural encounter with God, not just a method.

For more information on inner healing ministry from a Christian perspective, I highly recommend the late John Sandford's book *Deliverance and Inner Healing*. To find a healing minister, one good resource is the Elijah House Ministries website: https://www.elijahhouse.org/.

Some non-denominational charismatic and Pentecostal churches also have inner healing ministries. You don't necessarily have to be a member of these churches to receive ministry, and you can simply call and ask them if they offer inner healing prayer.

To learn more about sozo or theophostic ministry, visit the sites: BethelSozo.com and www.Theophostic.com.

Spiritual Oppression Causes Sleeplessness

It has been my personal experience that spiritual oppression is another major cause of insomnia, and of disease in general. I believe that we live in a world where the spiritual realm is more real than and superior to, the natural realm. The Bible teaches that evil spiritual entities do exist, and they can affect our lives, if we allow them to. Consider this verse from the book of Ephesians, Chapter 6, verse 12 in the Bible, "For we are not fighting against flesh-and-blood enemies, but against evil rulers and authorities of the unseen world, against mighty powers in this dark world, and against evil spirits in the heavenly places." (NLT).

This verse suggests that the real source of many of our problems isn't in the natural realm and is caused instead by evil spirits in the unseen world. I believe God has an agenda to share His love with the world through us, and that evil spiritual forces will throw up roadblocks to anyone who aligns with that agenda. Actually, we are all afflicted by evil, but the attacks upon those who have any kind of personal relationship with God may be even fiercer.

What's more, there are secret societies and cults worldwide that have malicious intentions and harness the power of evil spirits to harm to others. People in these societies take secret oaths and perform witchcraft-type rituals that bring curses such as insomnia upon their families (even extended families) and ancestors. Interestingly, people often join these cults with good intentions, and are even unaware that they have taken oaths or pronounced curses upon their families through their activities, because the process of indoctrination can be covert. And it happens more often than you might think.

Yet the curses occur because someone in the family history has sworn allegiance to an evil spiritual entity and pronounced curses over the generational line. I won't say much more about this topic, except to share my own experience, as I realize that the concept of spiritual oppression may be too "far out there" for some of you, or out of alignment with your religious beliefs. Yet I would like to briefly mention it because it has been my personal experience that many illnesses and conditions, including insomnia, are caused directly by oppression from evil spirits. I know because I have been used by God to set many people free from these conditions using deliverance prayer. Indeed, this is the only way to break free from insomnia that's caused by spiritual oppression.

The Power of Prayer for Removing Spiritual Causes of Insomnia

If you are interested in learning more about how God and prayer can set you free from spiritual oppression, I encourage you to listen to the Spiritual Principles for Wellness webinar series on my website, in which I teach about spiritual healing and how to break free from spiritual oppression and curses. For more information, see: http://conniestrasheim.org/webinars/. To learn more about how God heals supernaturally, I recommend my book, *Healing Chronic Illness: By His Spirit, Through His Resources.*

When my battle with insomnia was at its worst, I asked a group of people to pray for me everyday for a month. It was a huge request, but the battle had become so intense that I knew I needed outside help, because God had impressed it upon me that the war I was waging in my body wasn't just a biochemical one, but also a spiritual one. At the same time, I enlisted an experienced healing prayer minister whom I knew had a very developed and discerning spirit, to ask God what was hindering my healing in the spiritual realm. A few things emerged from my sessions with her.

First and foremost, she discerned that subconsciously, I associated sleep with death. I feared sleep because it meant that I might not exist anymore. On a conscious level, I didn't believe this, but because I had a traumatic birth and apparently my heart had stopped at some point during my delivery, there could have been trauma stored in my body from that experience which caused me associate sleep with dying.

Having been raised in an emotionally volatile home, I also learned to be hyper vigilant, so it may be that I did not feel that going to sleep was safe, because when you are asleep, you can't remain alert to protect yourself. So I worked with the prayer minister to heal those parts of me that didn't feel safe in the world.

The minister also discerned that there were generational curses in my family line that had caused me to become ill. I was a bit surprised to learn that I wasn't sleeping in part due to some curse that had been placed upon me by a family member or ancestor. But sure enough, after I worked with the healing minister for some time, I began to witness greater breakthroughs and acceleration in the restoration of my sleep patterns and an improvement in my overall wellbeing. In the end, I don't know how much of a role the emotional and spiritual factors played in my battle with insomnia, but I believe they were fairly significant because my journey toward wellness got easier and moved along much faster after that.

I would have never expected that emotional and spiritual issues were at the root of the sleep issues that I battled, but in the end, it turns out that they were part of the problem. Sometimes, by dealing with trauma and/or the emotional causes of insomnia, the spiritual causes of insomnia are automatically resolved, since trauma can open the door to spiritual oppression. Regardless of your beliefs, it's important address any past trauma and/or emotional issues in your life, as these may be playing a role in your inability to sleep.

Chapter Twelve

Tools for Weaning off of Benzodiazepines and Other Sleep Medications

One of the most difficult things that I've ever done, and paradoxically, one of the best decisions that I've ever made to regain my health, was to quit anti-depressant and benzodiazepine medications, after more than 10 years of on-again, off-again use.

While these drugs helped me in the short run to overcome depression, insomnia, and other symptoms that accompanied my battle with Lyme disease, over the long term, they worsened my symptoms. The turning point when I finally decided to quit all of them was when I realized that the benzodiazepine drug that I was taking, lorazepam, was damaging my memory and ability to reason and function cognitively. Lorazepam is one of the most addictive medications there is, so I won't lie—letting go of it was hard.

The weaning process took many months, and was fraught with withdrawal symptoms such as massive insomnia (one of the conditions that it was intended to treat), anxiety, chest pain, severe depression, heart palpitations, back pain, fatigue, hallucinations, mild seizures, shakiness, and more.

Had I known then what I know now about how to restore the brain and body during and after benzodiazepine and antidepressant use, I think the withdrawal process might have been much easier for me. If you are addicted to antidepressants, sedatives and/or other sleep meds, I want to encourage you that it is possible to get off of these medications and heal your brain with nutrients.

I believe there is a place for medication in the short-term; in emergency situations, and I judge nobody who takes them, but know this—in the long run, they will most likely harm your body in some way, and there are often better ways to manage your symptoms.

I will preface all this by saying that drug withdrawal is often not easy, and it's not a do-it-yourself endeavor. You need emotional and professional support, but that doesn't mean a doctor who tells you to taper off of your meds within just two weeks, or even a month. If you've been on sleep medication for more than a short period of time, which could be defined as anywhere from several months to several years, you may need many months, as in 6-8 months, or even longer, to wean off of them. And you'll want to work with a professional; an addictions counselor and/or medical doctor who really understands drug addiction. This is very important.

It took me two years to fully wean off of the antidepressant and benzodiazepine medications, and perhaps two more years to really heal my brain and body from the effects of those medications (and I am still healing, in fact). But again, I believe that I can help to shorten the runway for you with some of the tools that I share here. Feel free to share these with your doctor.

I have found all of the following to help me recover from anti-depressant and sedative withdrawal/addiction:

- Amino acid therapy (especially GABA, 5-HTP and L-tyrosine). Sedatives act as a potent type of artificial GABA in the body, so taking supplemental GABA can help to make the transition off of these kinds of drugs a bit easier. 5-HTP and L-tyrosine can help to improve symptoms of insomnia, brain fog, depression, fatigue and other symptoms that are commonly caused by drug withdrawal, and in the long run, are good replacements for antidepressant medication.

- Brain wave entrainment therapy. This is especially useful for treating "rebound insomnia" which occurs as a part of sleep medication withdrawal.

- Hormonal and nutritional support. The better your diet is, the lesser will be the effects of any drug withdrawal symptoms. I highly recommend reading Lee Cowden, MDs and my 2014 book, *Foods that Fit a Unique You* for more information on a healthy, anti-inflammatory diet that can be tailored to your specific needs

- Prayer. God works in supernatural ways and can sustain you above and beyond what you are able to do in the natural realm. I could not have endured drug withdrawal without the support of God and the prayers of others. Consider joining a faith-based community and enlisting the help of at least several prayer partners as you go through the drug withdrawal process.

- Emotional support. You'll need at least one friend that you can call at any hour of the day, when you are going through difficult withdrawal symptoms. I was grateful to be able to awaken my sweetheart Bill at 2 or 3 AM whenever the insomnia, depression and/or other symptoms became unbearable. He often encouraged, consoled and prayed for me, which enabled me to endure and keep on going. Support groups can also be helpful.

- A competent medical doctor and/or addictions counselor, who can help you to determine how you should taper off your medications and monitor you as you go through the process

- Getting enough sunshine and making sure that you take care of your soul's needs. Do something daily that brings you joy, such as watching an uplifting television program, reading a good novel, or simply spending some time daily in nature or with friends.

- Exercise, which helps your body to heal on multiple levels.

This information is only meant to be a starting point, to give you a broad idea about some of the tools that are sometimes needed to effectively withdraw and heal from the effects of sleep medication addiction. In most cases, an arsenal of tools is required, but it *is* possible, if not easy, to get off of these drugs. Just don't do it quickly, and don't do it on your own, especially if you have been taking the medication(s) for more than a few months.

For more information on how to withdraw from benzodiazepines, I highly recommend the book, *Recovery and Renewal: Your Essential Guide to Overcoming Dependency and Withdrawal from Sleeping Pills, Other 'Benzo' Tranquillisers and Antidepressants* by addictions counselor Baylissa Frederick. Dr. Frederick also does personal Skype consultations, for anyone who is interested. For more information, visit her website: https://baylissa.com/.

Chapter Thirteen

Stack Your Sleep Solutions, and Put Together a Plan to Make It all Work Together

If you're like I was, and your insomnia is due to multiple factors, including neurodegenerative disease, trauma and a poor sleep environment, you may find that no one single supplement, tool or other remedy will be enough to full restore your sleep. You may need to do or take three, four or five different things. Or, you may find one tool that is so powerful that it covers the most important bases—which would be great!

I share this because I don't want you to get discouraged if you find that one tool or remedy isn't enough to get you a full eight hours (or whatever you may need) of shut-eye at night. Chances are, you will either need a different tool, more than one tool, or simply some time for your body to re-calibrate and re-adjust to the changes. Sometimes, the process is fast; at other times, it takes weeks or months to reap the full benefits of the tools.

It took me several years to fully normalize and restore my sleep after battling severe insomnia for nearly a decade. It may take your body some time, too, but your healing runway is likely to be much shorter than mine if you use the tools that I provide in this book, as it took me years and a lot of experimentation to learn about all of them. Nonetheless, it can still take many weeks, or months, to fully restore your body if you have battled sleeplessness for years.

The other reason it may take some time to heal is because most likely, you'll need to experiment with some of the solutions in this book to find those that will best work for you. Most of the tools here can be used simultaneously, and "stacked" one on top of the other, but I strongly urge you to only try out one at a time, to gauge your response to that tool before adding to it or moving on to another. You'll also want to ask your doctor whether any of the remedies or tools mentioned in this book conflict with any medications or other supplements that you are taking. This is important. In general, everything that I recommend here is safe for most people, but we are all different, and not everyone responds well to the same things.

What to do First and Tips for Putting Together a Plan that Works for You

As a first step to resolving insomnia, I highly recommend lowering the amount of electromagnetic pollution in your environment and practicing proper sleep hygiene. We are all negatively impacted by the multitude of manmade electromagnetic fields (EMFs) in our environment, and chances are, EMFs are impacting your body's chemistry, whether you feel it or not. As I mentioned earlier, thousands have studies have proven that EMFs are a major cause of insomnia, cancer, neurodegenerative disease and many other conditions, so shielding yourself from EMFs is simply a good idea.

I have found EMFs to be one of those stealth toxins that nobody thinks is keeping them awake at night but which is actually a major cause of insomnia in many people. So even if you can't afford to buy EMF shielding for your bed or Graham-Stetzer filters, at least turn off the appliances and/or circuit breakers in your bedroom at night, along with your cell phone, wireless router and cordless phones. If this doesn't help to resolve your insomnia, and EMF testing indicates that you are still bathing in a field of high frequencies, you will want to consider investing in some EMF-protection products.

Just as unplugging the appliances in your bedroom at night and turning off your cell phone and circuit breakers costs nothing, so does proper sleep hygiene, which will also help to encourage restful sleep. Again, it is important to go to bed and get up at the same time daily, as this will help you to establish a healthy circadian rhythm in your body. Even if you can't seem to get to sleep or get up at the same hour, do your best to maintain a consistent sleep schedule.

To facilitate this, you might practice doing quiet activities before bedtime, rather than being on your computer, cell phone or other stimulating devices that can keep you awake. It may be hard at first to change any long-engrained habits of working late, or checking Facebook or your email before bedtime, but I think you will find that it's well worth the effort.

If practicing proper sleep hygiene and cleaning up the electromagnetic pollution in your environment isn't enough to get you to sleep, as a next step, you may want to get your hormones and neurotransmitters tested, especially if you suffer from a neurological health condition or are a woman over 35. Your doctor can then recommend supplements or medications that will help you to balance your chemistry, based on your test results.

Or, you might simply ask your doctor about trying out some amino acids such as GABA or 5HTP, or even melatonin, to see if these supplements help you to sleep. I don't like taking supplements without doing a test first to see what I need, as it's sort of a "hit or miss" way to treat sleep problems, but the reality is, I understand that many of you may not have the financial resources to spend on testing in order to discover every underlying cause of your insomnia. But know this—you can end up wasting a lot of time and money on "hit or miss" treatments if you don't do testing to determine what's keeping you up at night, and such treatments (even if they are natural) can occasionally be harmful.

Next, if you have a chronic illness or other symptoms besides insomnia, I recommend having your doctor test you to determine whether inflammation and/or mast cell activation disorder (MCAD) are an underlying cause of your insomnia. If so, you'll want to consider solutions for lowering the inflammation in your body. You may be surprised at how many people don't sleep due to inflammation.

Solutions for inflammation include, first and foremost, maintaining an anti-inflammatory diet and addressing the causes of inflammation, which commonly include: infections, stress, and environmental toxins. In addition, you may find natural or prescription anti-inflammatory remedies to be important.

When you are deciding upon which sleep tools will be most effective for you, it's important to consider whether you have more trouble falling asleep at night, or awaken frequently, or awaken too early in the morning. Do you have nightmares or night terrors? Do you take your problems to bed with you at night? All of these will factor into the type of tools that you'll want to use to get better and more long-lasting shut-eye.

First, if you have difficulty falling asleep, consider whether you are taking your worries to bed with you. If so, your first line of treatment should be to focus on the mind-body relaxation and spiritual strategies for sleep described in this book.

Also, you may have trouble falling asleep if your cortisol levels are too high at night, or you have too high levels of glutamate, an excitatory neurotransmitter found in excess in people with neurotoxin syndromes. Your body may also be inflamed (when your cortisol levels are too high, you will tend to have inflammation) and/or your other hormones and neurotransmitters may be out of balance.

If this is the case, you'll want to get your hormones and neurotransmitters tested, and then have your doctor prescribe the proper supplements and/or pharmaceutical remedies to balance those out. If you awaken periodically throughout the night, this can also be caused by hormone and neurotransmitter imbalances.

Another great tool to use if you have trouble falling asleep are brain wave entrainment devices such as the sound-light machine. I have found these to work better for helping people to fall asleep, rather than for going back to sleep in the middle of the night or early morning. They are also helpful for withdrawing from sleep medication, and for helping the mind to release worries before bedtime.

If you are able to fall asleep at night, but awaken too early in the morning, consider taking cannabis or amino acids such as GABA, 5-HTP or theanine to help you fall back asleep. Chances are, these will leave you less groggy the next day than other sleep supplements and medications. For instance, melatonin is best taken right before bedtime, rather than in the early morning, as it can leave you groggy the next day. That said, we are unique and respond differently to different things. One person may be able to take GABA at 5 AM, sleep for a few hours, and feel great the next day, while another may only be able to take GABA in small doses at bedtime, or not at all.

Another great strategy that I have found that helps me to go back to sleep when I awaken too early in the morning is to have a small bowl of gluten-free oatmeal with some butter and cinnamon (cinnamon helps to balance the blood sugar). Oatmeal contains tryptophan, which is a precursor to serotonin, a calming neurotransmitter that aids in sleep.

If you awaken at the same time every night, it may be a clue that one of your organs is stressed, because each of the organs' energy is strongest during a particular time of night. So if you have a problem in a particular organ, you may awaken during the hours when that organ's energy is at its highest. For example, if you awaken between 1-3 AM, when the liver and gallbladder are most active detoxifying your body, it may be that these organs are being overloaded from processing toxins. If you discover that to be true, you'll want to ask your doctor about doing some detoxification treatments to help facilitate the removal of those toxins or support those organs.

Or, for instance, if you awaken around 5-6 AM, your blood sugar may be low and your adrenal function inadequate. If this is the case, consider having a protein snack at bedtime. At times throughout my recovery, I have needed to eat animal protein before bedtime; a chicken leg, or beef stick, in order to sleep eight solid hours. A handful of nuts or a wimpy vegetarian protein powder drink just wouldn't cut it for me. You may find the same to be true for you.

Finally, consider spiritual counseling and ministry, or limbic system retraining using a program such as DNRS, if the biochemical tools that I have shared in this book aren't enough. I actually recommend emotional healing strategies as a first line of treatment for anyone who has a history of trauma, especially if the trauma was severe or prolonged, since traumatic memories and a limbic system that's stuck in "fight or flight" mode can play a major role in insomnia.

Research shows that insomnia is a common manifestation of depression, and that by getting healed from the depression, you can more easily resolve the insomnia. My 2019 book, *Healthy, Happy and Free: Spirit-Soul-Body Solutions for Healing from Depression* contains some great tools on how to heal from depression, which you may find to be helpful if you suspect depression to be a cause of your insomnia.

Consider also that some tools, such as the sound-light brain wave device, can address multiple causes of insomnia. This is because, for instance, when you normalize your brain waves, you also normalize your body's chemistry, while also calming your mind and nervous system. Some brain wave entrainment devices, such as the Neurointegrator by Clear Mind, can also help to alleviate depression and anxiety.

Antihistamines and anti-inflammatory remedies can sometimes also cover multiple bases as well, as when you lower inflammation in your body, your hormones and other chemicals such as cortisol, will also tend to normalize. Addressing mast cell activation and/or other histamine disorders can help your body to function better on many levels, which in turn, will help you to sleep. Of course, it's also essential to address the *root cause* of mast cell activation and inflammation, which can be mold toxicity, stress, Lyme disease and/or other infections, as well as other factors.

Other sleep tools will be more useful for addressing specific problems. For instance, if you have hypothyroidism or adrenal fatigue, you'll want to support your adrenal glands and thyroid with the proper nutrients or thyroid hormone replacement therapy.

You may find that uncovering the root causes of your insomnia is not a straightforward process, and that even once you do know why you can't sleep or aren't getting enough sleep, finding the proper treatment is somewhat of a trial and error process.

What's more, your body may or may not respond well to taking multiple remedies or using multiple tools at once, and you'll have to be patient with the "stacking" process. Further, it may take your body some time to heal and re-calibrate if you have been battling insomnia for a long time, so don't give up if one of the tools doesn't work right away, or only improves things gradually, or by degrees. Patience is important in this process!

In any case, please don't give up, as sometimes the healing process is two steps forward, one step back. On the other hand, you just may be one of those lucky ones who will find what you need right away, and that your sleep will normalize immediately. In any case, if you have been battling insomnia for months, or years, take heart—you can get better! Again, it may take you some time to discover those tools that will work best for you, but with perseverance, I believe that you will find them and will be well on your way to better sleep!

In Summary

The arsenal of tools that I have shared with you throughout this book include:

- **Remediating your home environment for electromagnetic pollution**

  This involves, in a nutshell:

  1. Turning off the circuit breakers and unplugging all electrical appliances in your bedroom at night
  2. Turning off all Wi-Fi, cell phones and cordless phones
  3. Using EMF shielding products such as Graham-Stetzer filters and EMF sleep canopies
  4. Moving your bedroom to another room, or moving to another location, if the EMFs are too high to be remediated

- **Practicing proper sleep hygiene**

  This involves such things as:

  1. Getting off your computer and cell phone and avoiding all "glowing gadgets" within two hours before bedtime
  2. Going to bed and getting up at the same time every day

3. Exposing yourself to bright sunlight within an hour of arising
4. Doing quiet, peaceful and relaxing activities before bedtime. This may include listening to meditative audio CDs, taking a hot bath, doing a sauna and/or lying on a Biomat, or reading a good book.
5. Doing light exercise during the day, which will help you to sleep at night

*   **Testing for and fixing any neurotransmitter imbalances**

Some tools for this include:

1. Taking amino acids such as GABA, taurine, theanine, 5-HTP and tryptophan, which relax the nervous system and increase serotonin
2. Taking methylation supplements to aid in neurotransmitter synthesis. These include nutrients such as: SAM-e, methyl-folate, P5P and Vitamin B-12.
3. Taking oxaloacetate to lower glutamate, an excitatory neurotransmitter that causes wakefulness

- **Testing and treating any hormonal imbalances**

Some tools for doing this include:

1. Vitamin C, pantethine, rhodiola, licorice root, ashwaghanda, and adrenal glandular formulas for adrenal fatigue/insufficiency
2. Bio-identical hormones such as pregnenolone, 7-keto DHEA, DHEA, progesterone and cortisol (among others, as test results indicate)
3. Phosphatidylserine to lower high nighttime cortisol levels
4. Iodine, selenium and bio-identical thyroid hormone to correct thyroid abnormalities
5. An anti-inflammatory diet which includes foods in their natural state that are organic and low glycemic, especially vegetables, fruits, healthy fats and animal protein

- **Lowering inflammation and histamine, and treating mast cell activation disorder (MCAD) with:**

1. Ketitofen and other anti-histamine medications
2. Natural remedies such as quercetin and diamine oxidase
3. Supplements that support healthy histamine levels, such as Siberian ginseng, Vitamin C, magnesium glycinate, and holy basil
4. Curcumin, omega-3 essential fatty acids and other anti-inflammatory remedies
5. Following an anti-histamine diet

- **Balancing your brain waves and calming your nervous system with entrainment therapies**

  These include:

  1. Neurofeedback devices such as those from Clear Mind
  2. Light-Sound machines, such as those from Tools for Wellness

- **Treating pain and helping your body to relax** with cannabis and menthol-based ointments, Epsom salt baths and/or a Biomat

- **Addressing the emotional and spiritual causes of insomnia**

  Some tools that I recommend for this include:

  1. Inner healing prayer, to heal the effects of past or current traumas that may be impacting your sleep
  2. Counseling, to heal past or current traumas that may be impacting your sleep
  3. Guided relaxation or meditative CDs or MP3 downloads
  4. Practicing surrender and giving your fears over to God
  5. Using reframing techniques to fill your mind with positive truths, to replace fear-based thinking
  6. Using mind-body strategies to heal the limbic system, emotions and body. Some tools that are useful for this include:
     a) Dynamic Neural Retraining (DNRS)
     b) The King Method (TKM)

c) Inner healing prayer systems such as SOZO and Theophostic

7. Getting up and doing an activity that will help you to take your mind off of yours fears of not sleeping

8. Enlisting the help of an addictions counselor, medical doctor or other qualified health care practitioner to help you wean off of sleep medication (if needed)

- **Taking other sleep supplements, which may include:**

1. Cannabis, which is very calming and healing to the nervous system

2. Melatonin, which helps to establish a healthy sleep-wake cycle

3. Herbal remedies such as Valerian root, chamomile, passionflower and lavender, which also aid in relaxation

4. Homeopathic sleep remedies that are specific to the type of sleep problems that you have

I hope you have found this short, succinct book on insomnia to be helpful for you! It does not cover every single solution for sleeplessness, only those that I have personally found to be most beneficial and which I know others with neurological illness or other chronic health conditions have found to be helpful. Undoubtedly, there are other great resources out there that provide other solutions in addition to those described here, and I encourage you to do further research on your own, if need be, to aid you in your healing journey.

In the meantime, I believe that if you will faithfully give a few of the tools in this book a try, you will find yourself sleeping longer and better than you ever have before. Be patient with the process—it may take time for your brain and body to recover and reprogram itself from any damage done by infections, trauma, toxins and other factors, but I believe that if you persevere, you will eventually recover and find healing from chronic sleep deprivation. May you be blessed in your healing journey!

Additional References and Resources

Chapter Two: Revitalize Your Sleep by Removing Electromagnetic Pollution from Your Home

Books and Scientific Articles/Reports

Gittelman, Ann Louise. 2011. *Zapped: Why Your Cell Phone Shouldn't Be Your Alarm Clock and 1,268 Ways to Outsmart the Hazards of Electronic Pollution.* Harper One; Reprint edition.

Rees, Camilla. 2009. *Public Health SOS: The Shadow Side Of The Wireless Revolution.* Create Space.

The Bio Initiative Report 2012. *The BioInitiative Working Group.* Accessed on February 13, 2017 from: BioInitiative.org.

EMF Measuring Devices and Shielding Products

Cornet ED78S EMF RF Electrosmog meter. Available at LessEMF.com, Amazon and other online retailers.

Electromagnetic Shielding Material. EMF Safety Store: EMFsafetystore.com/#fabric.

Graham-Stetzer filters: StetzerElectric.com or Stetzerizer-US.com.

Grounding Products: The Earthing Institute: EarthingInstitute.net and Earthing.com.

Swiss Shield Naturell bed canopy. EMF Safety Store: EMFSafetyStore.com/#canopies.

The EMF Safety Shop: LessEMF.com
The EMF Safety Store: EMFSafetyStore.com.

The International Institute for Building Biology and Ecology: http://hbelc.org/find-an-expert/environmental-consultants.

Chapter Three: Sleep Deeper by Lowering Histamine and Inflammation

Books and Articles

Afrin, L. 2016. *Never Bet Against Occam: Mast Cell Activation Disease and the Modern Epidemics of Chronic Illness and Medical Complexity*. Sisters Media, LLC; 1 edition.

Strasheim, Connie. 2016. *New Paradigms in Lyme Disease Treatment: 10 Top Doctors Reveal Healing Strategies that Work*. S. Lake Tahoe: BioMed Publishing Group. For more information, see: www.NewLymeTreatments.com.

Tsafrir, J. Histamine Intolerance, GAPS and Low Carb. February 21, 2013. *JudyTsafrirMD.com*. Accessed on February 13, 2017 from: JudyTsafrirMD.com.

Products
benaGene. Terra Biological, LLC: Benagene.com.

Bosmeric-SR (patented blend of curcumin): Bosmeric-SR.com.
Cereze, by Sabre Sciences:
SabreSciences.com/store/CEREZE
Ketotifen – Key Pharmacy: KeyCompounding.com.

Gene, Amino Acid and Neurotransmitter Testing

Sabre Sciences: SabreSciences.com
NeuroScience: WhyNeuroScience.com
Pharmasan: Pharmasan.com
BioHealth Diagnostics: BioHealthLab.com
23 and me gene testing: 23andme.com

Amino Acid Products

Kavinace and Kavinace Ultra PM, by NeuroScience:
NeuroScienceInc.com.

Chapter Five: Modulate Your Brain Waves with Entrainment Therapy

Books

Bowthorpe, J. 2011. *Stop the Thyroid Madness: A Patient Revolution Against Decades of Inferior Treatment.* Laughing Grape Publishing.

Kharrazian, Datis. DHSc, DC, MS. 2010. *Why Do I Still Have Thyroid Symptoms when My Lab Tests Are Normal: a Revolutionary Breakthrough in Understanding Hashimoto's Disease and Hypothyroidism.* Elephant Press; 1st edition.

Lam, M. 2012. *Adrenal Fatigue: - Reclaim Your Energy and Vitality with Clinically Proven Natural Programs.* Adrenal Institute Press.

Strasheim, Connie and Cowden, W. Lee. 2014. *BioEnergetic Tools for Wellness.* ACIM Press.

Products

Light and Sound Machines. Tools for Wellness: ToolsForWellness.com

Neurointegrator neurofeedback device. Clear Mind Center: ClearMindCenter.com.

Chapter Six: Balance Your Hormones with Natural Supplements and Bio-Identical Hormone Replacement Therapy

Books

Bowthorpe, J. 2011. *Stop the Thyroid Madness: A Patient Revolution Against Decades of Inferior Treatment.* Laughing Grape Publishing.

Lam, M. 2012. *Adrenal Fatigue - Reclaim Your Energy and Vitality with Clinically Proven Natural Programs.* Adrenal Institute Press.

Northrup, C. 2010. *Women's Bodies, Women's Wisdom: Creating Physical and Emotional Health and Healing.* Bantam; Rev Upd edition (June 1, 2010)

Pollen, M. 2009. *Food Rules: An Eater's Manual.* Penguin Books; 1st edition.

Strasheim, Connie. 2012. *Beyond Lyme Disease: Healing the Underlying Causes of Chronic Illness in those with Borreliosis and Co-Infections.* S. Lake Tahoe: BioMed Publishing Group.

Strasheim, Connie and Cowden, W. Lee. 2014. *Foods that Fit a Unique You.* ACIM Press.

Adrenal Glandular Products

Adrenal Dessicated: StandardProcess.com
ADB5 Plus: BioticsResearch.com.

Where to Find an Integrative Medical Doctor

Academy for Comprehensive Integrative Medicine (ACIM): ACIMConnect.com.
American College for Advancement in Medicine (ACAM): ACAM.org.
The Institute for Functional Medicine: FunctionalMedicine.org
Cholesterol from New Beginnings: nbnus.net.

Chapter Seven: Rest Better by Removing Pain and Chronic Infections

Mediflow water pillow: Mediflow.com.

SAMINA mattresses: JustHealthySleep.com/sleeping-systems/

Cannabis Products

Bluebird Botanicals CBD oil: Bluebird-botanicals.com

Mary's Medicinals CBD/CBN and THC based products: MarysMedicinals.com/products

Other Pain Remedies

Sombra pain gel: SombraUSA.com
Biomat: Biomat.com.

Books

Strasheim, Connie and Cowden, W. Lee. 2014. *Create a Toxin-Free Body or Home...Starting Today.* ACIM Press.

Chapter Eight: Relax Your Body and Mind with Cannabis and Botanical and Homeopathic Remedies

Books and Articles

Curtin, D. "Sleep Problems." British Homeopathic Association: BritishHomeopathic.org.

Products

Babuna and Amantilla NutraMedix products: NutraMedix.com.

Chapter Nine: Discover the King Method®: a Free Hands-On Healing Tool

King, G. The King Method®: KingInstitute.org.
King, G. TKM Median Sequence:
https://www.kinginstitute.org/attachments/article/319/M
EDIAN%20Seq..pdf

Chapter Ten: Practice Proper Sleep Hygiene with Healthy Nighttime Habits

Frederick, B. 2014. *Recovery and Renewal: Your Essential Guide to Overcoming Dependency and Withdrawal from Sleeping Pills, Other 'Benzo' Tranquillisers and Antidepressants.* Jessica Kingsley; Revised edition edition (May 21, 2014).

Chapter Eleven: Heal from the Emotional and Spiritual Causes of Insomnia

Books and Audio Resources

Hopper, A. Dynamic Neural Retraining (DNRT): RetrainingtheBrain.com.

King, G. The King Method (TKM): KingInstitute.org.

Meditative and Audio CDs: Insomnia.net: Insomnia.net/natural-remedies/cds/

Sanford, J.2008. *Deliverance and Inner Healing.* Chosen Books; Revised ed. edition

Strasheim, Connie. Spiritual Principles for Wellness webinar series, 2014: http://conniestrasheim.org/webinars/.

Strasheim, C. 2010. *Healing Chronic Illness: By His Spirit, Through His Resources.* S. Lake Tahoe: BioMed Publishing Group.

Inner Healing Ministry Resources:

Elijah House Ministries: ElijahHouse.org
SOZO: BethelSozo.com
Theophostic Ministry: Theophostic.com.

Endnotes

[i] Do we know enough to take action? BioInitiative Report 2012: A Rationale for Biologically Based Exposure Standards for Low-Intensity Electromagnetic Radiation. *BioInitiative Working Group*. Accessed on Feb. 7, 2017 from: http://www.bioinitiative.org/participants/do-we-know-enough-to-take-action/

[ii] Afrin, L. 2016. *Never Bet Against Occam: Mast Cell Activation Disease and the Modern Epidemics of Chronic Illness and Medical Complexity*, Sister's Media, LLC.

[iii] Pai, S. The Truth About Cancer documentary, 2016, Ty and Charlene Bollinger.

[iv] Tsafrir, J. Histamine Intolerance, GAPS and Low Carb. *Judy Tsafrir, MD.com*. Feb. 21, 2013. Accessed on February 13, 2017 from: http://www.judytsafrirmd.com/

[v] Zlotnik A1, Gruenbaum SE, Artru AA, Rozet I, Dubilet M, Tkachov S, Brotfain E, Klin Y, Shapira Y, Teichberg VI. The neuroprotective effects of oxaloacetate in closed head injury in rats is mediated by its blood glutamate scavenging activity: evidence from the use of maleate. *J Neurosurg Anesthesiol*. 2009 Jul;21(3):235-41. doi: 10.1097/ANA.0b013e3181a2bf0b.

[vi] Gottlieb M1, Wang Y, Teichberg VI. Blood-mediated scavenging of cerebrospinal fluid glutamate . J Neurochem. (2003) Oct;87(1):119-26.

[vii] Ripps, S. Review: Taurine: a 'very essential' amino acid. *Mol Vis*. 18:2673-86 (2012).

[viii] [viii] Rog DJ1, Nurmikko TJ, Friede T, Young CA. Randomized, controlled trial of cannabis-based medicine in central pain in multiple sclerosis. *Neurology*. 2005 Sep 27;65(6):812-9

Discover Other Books by Connie Strasheim at:

ConnieStrasheim.org

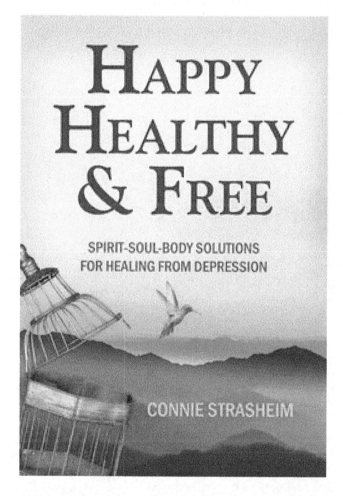

Combines wisdom on divine healing and natural
medicine to bring you better answers for healing
from depression, in spirit, soul and body!

For more information on Bill Gonseaux's book, see:

TheGodWhoLovesMe.com

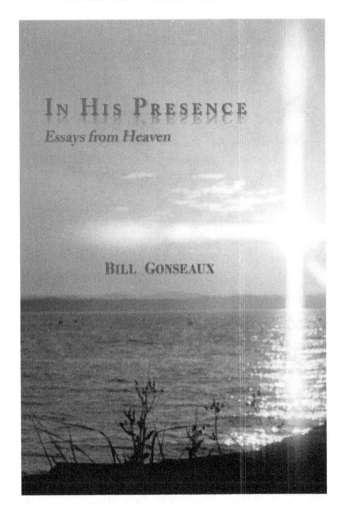

Made in the USA
Coppell, TX
19 June 2022

79025063R00079